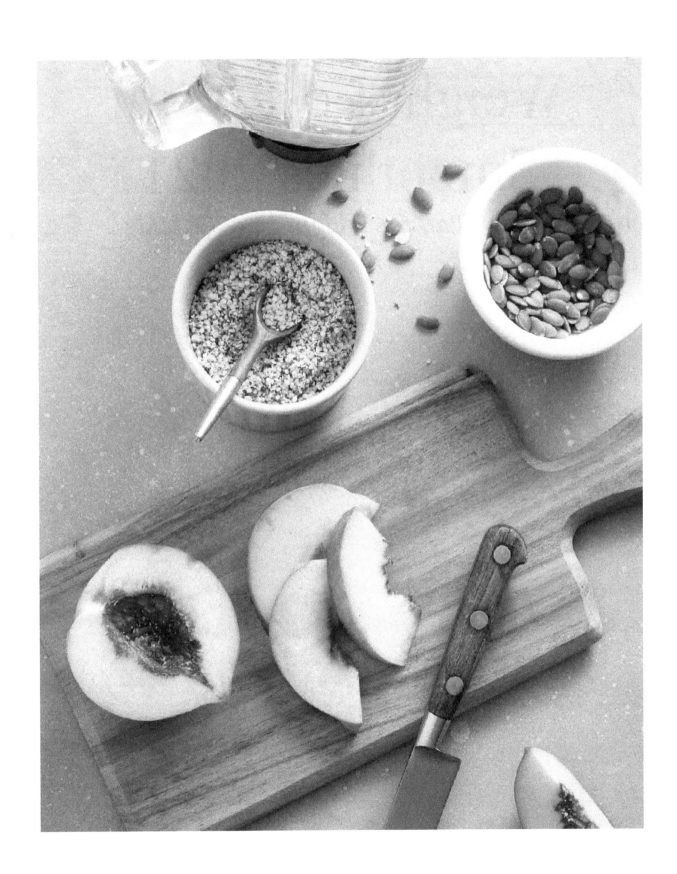

Weight Lose With Smoothies 2021

A Day Plan for Weight Lose Quickly

Contents

The Wise Watermelon
Cherries Joybilee
The Green Berry Banana
Cherry Charlie Checker
Bear's Choice
Rosy-Red Robin
Pom Dot Com
Rainbow Bright
The Three Bears
Tropical Storm Theo
Nutty Nittany Lion
Alf's Apple Pie
Strawberry Summer 365
The Pretty Peach
Raspberry Rocks
Wholly Melon
Sweet Tater
Cherry Michele Chanel
Macho Green Matcha
The Vitamin C Note
Eddie B's Monday-Morning Doubles
Zurprise!
Banana Buddhaberry
Naked Nut-trition
The Sammer Jammer
It's Cocopletely Bananas
Patty Papaya
Minty Makeover
Jerry's Purple Jam
The Baked Big Apple
Classic Creamsicle

Metabolic Machine

Ahhh-mazing Acai

Not Yo Mama's Matcha

Keri's Berries

Eye of the Pumpkin

JP's Green Garden

Al's Iced Hazelnut

Workout Wonder

Cup of Joe Schmo

Grateful Green

The Bold Lip

The Waterlemon

Hirsch's Kiss

Wind Me Up

Salty Peanut Butter Pretzel

Sabrina's Spicy A.M. Shake-Up

The Superfruit Edition

Pop Pop's Parrothead Piña Colada

The GG (Great Green)

Mama's Milkshake

Banana Splitz

LB's Blissed-Out Berries

Pep in Your Step

Hair of the Dewy Dog

Red Tango

Dr. Jeff's Cardiac Cocktail

Becky's Afterburn Boost

Raspberry Rainy Day

Lola's Lemonade Stand

Anna's Bananas

Cha-Cha Cherry Chai

Matcha Average Avocado

Happy Holidaze

Frozen Peanut Butter Hot Cocoa

Secret Garden Smoothie

Strawberry Shanny and Friends

Roslyn Berry Blowout

Nat's Nutty by Nature

Kale 'Em with Kindness

Orange You Glad (This Is the Last Smoothie)!

Introduction

We all often feel overwhelmed with the general chaos of everyday life and the last thing we want to stress about is food. But we do all the time. So, get excited to incorporate smoothies into your diet, which will lead you down the path to a healthier you.

Before we begin, I want to tell you a little bit about my smoothie history, how I became a number one fan, and why I am so thrilled to teach you about them. I have been a proud smoothie lover for as long as I've been interested in food and nutrition (which is basically since I can recollect). I started my journey at a young age, so it makes sense that experimenting with smoothies is my top recommendation for parents to encourage their kids to get interested in health, too. With just a simple blender, anyone can enjoy throwing different ingredients together to create a colorful masterpiece. Smoothies meet my top four criteria—yummy, one container, nutritious, and quick—for creating a healthier, saner existence. When a meal actually helps you get out the door faster in the morning, tastes great, and makes you instantly feel awesome, then of course it becomes a staple of your diet. Having only one container to rinse seals the deal for me. Less prep and cleaning? Yes and yes.

I know, nutritionists and smoothies are so cliché. But we have good reason to recommend them! For the past 16 years, I have been creating meal plans for my clients that cover every age range and food preference, and I have always included smoothie recipes. The versatility of ingredients makes them chock-full of nutrition and they're an amazing way to increase variety in your diet for even the pickiest eaters. Just think about it: Into almost every smoothie, you can sneak powerhouse foods such as greens and seeds that you may not otherwise eat on their own, and you will never even know they're blended up into a tasty shake. The ingredients and superfood boosters are endless. Plus, as you get to know me, you will see how I like to throw together the easiest meals and I always have fun doing it. Let's make food fun again!

From the outside, food and nutrition appear more complicated than ever, but the truth is, they can be simple (and really enjoyable) if you approach them from a different point of view. I teach my clients to appreciate how nourishing, real foods can make your body work most efficiently from the inside out. There is no quick fix to changing your health and it takes time and patience, but doing the work becomes the shortcut. When you modify your habits into healthier ones, this way of life becomes second nature and the cycle of endless restrictive dieting will vanish. My mission is for you to live in the best of both food worlds by eating mostly real, nutritious foods as well as your favorites (without the guilt!). When the balance begins to naturally happen, you start to feel and look your best without the constant struggle.

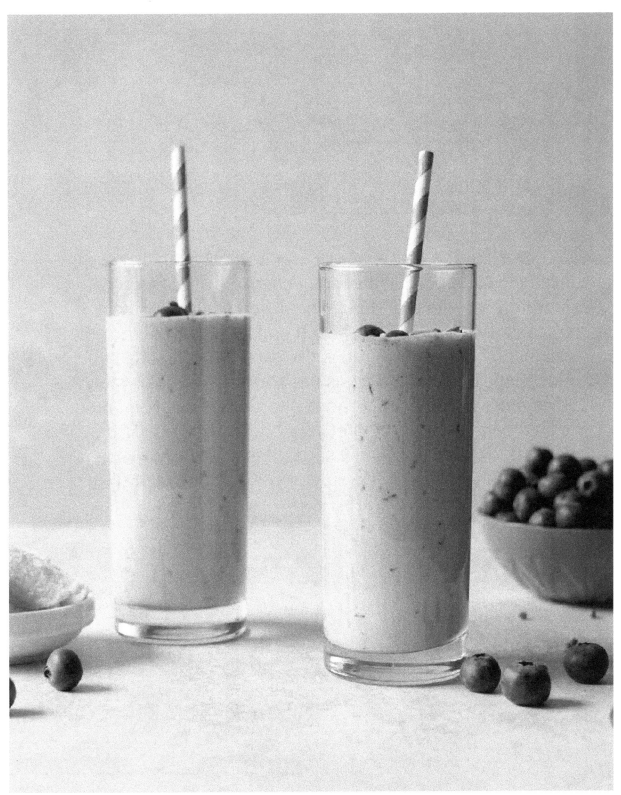

Big Blue

Chapter One
SLIM DOWN
ESSENTIALS

BEFORE WE BEGIN BLENDING, let's talk all things prep, including the smoothie creation essentials and, even more important, how to ease into mentally committing to the process of improving your health and moving closer to your weight goal. Smoothie prep is the easy part because even though the ingredient options are endless, you really only need a blender and a few staples to get started. Mind prep is a different story, but forget your past struggles and move forward. You are absolutely capable of positive, consistent health changes, so believe in yourself and let's kick off this journey together as a team. Follow along as I teach you how to become a smoothie-making master!

WHY SMOOTHIES?

Diet trends have shifted throughout the years, but smoothies will always stand the test of time as a super-quick, nutrient-dense meal or snack option. With just a few standard ingredients and a blender, you can create a tasty, filling meal that checks all the boxes on my nutrition barometer. The endless options for ingredients in a smoothie can easily satisfy the three macronutrients (carbohydrates, proteins, and fats) your body requires in a single glass. Meals are most complete when they combine fiber from complex carbohydrates with lean protein and quality fats, and smoothies are one of the most efficient ways to achieve this combo. They include a variety of nutrients that both mentally and physiologically satisfy your needs. This trifecta of nutrients slows digestion and keeps your blood sugar stable, which, in turn, satiates you longer. In order to adopt healthier eating habits that eventually become second nature, it is important to fill your diet with flavorful, satisfying, go-to meals, and smoothies fit that bill. One or two smoothies a day can be a realistic and effective approach to moving toward—and eventually meeting—your health and weight-loss goals.

VERSATILITY: SMOOTHIES ARE FOR EVERYONE

Whether you have food allergies, follow a medically restricted diet, or just prefer a certain approach to eating (as in a plant-based or vegan diet), smoothies are so versatile that they can be adjusted to meet any individual's dietary needs and preferences. Ingredients are easily "swappable," and the varieties of flavor combinations are endless. You can vary your smoothie picks based on the climate and temperature where you live, the season, local produce availability, workout routines, fluctuating schedules, food preferences, mood, or cravings. There is a smoothie for every appetite.

NUTRIENT-, ANTIOXIDANT-DENSE FOR HEALTHY WEIGHT LOSS

Smoothies represent basic Nutrition 101 as the ultimate example of a complete nutrient- and antioxidant-rich meal that fits into any healthy diet. The base of a smoothie usually includes fruits and vegetables, which are lacking in most American diets but are the ideal source of naturally occurring vitamins, minerals, and antioxidants. Smoothies are not only calorically appropriate for weight loss and/or healthy maintenance, but they are also full of health benefits. By replacing processed meals and snack foods with smoothies, you can decrease your consumption of added sugar, unhealthy fats, and sodium while bumping up fiber and nutrient intake significantly. As a mom and nutrition counselor of sometimes-picky eaters, smoothies are my first pick when it comes to fitting more fresh foods into limited diets. By blending fruits and leafy greens (like kale and spinach) with heart-healthy proteins and fat (like avocado and seeds), you can enjoy a nutritious meal disguised in a tasty blended shake. The ingredients are so variable in smoothies that you can easily consume a wide variety of nutrients by making simple swaps.

SMOOTHIES SAVE TIME

Quick and easy is the name of the game when it comes to maintaining a healthy diet. My clients require simplicity in their meal prep. Our busy lives don't leave much time to shop for food and prepare complicated meals, but with just a couple of staple ingredients, anyone can whip up a nutritious, complete meal in minutes. A standard smoothie includes fruits and/or veggies (which I typically buy frozen so they last and create frostiness without the need for ice cubes); a protein option such as yogurt, protein powder, or nut/seed butter; and a form of liquid such as milk or water to blend it all together. Plus, they're tough to mess up because you can easily follow the recipe and then adjust for taste and texture preferences. With the push of a button, you've suddenly created a healthy meal that really feels like a treat. If you drink smoothies, you already know they instantly make you feel healthier and more energized after just a few sips.

GET YOUR MIND RIGHT

I hate to break it to you, but restrictive diets don't work. I bet you know this because you've already tried plenty of them and you end up in a worse place than where you started. Fad diets are temporary fixes that don't actually address the core problems you are struggling with in your life, like stress, hormonal imbalances, inadequate sleep and fatigue, lack of nutrition education, or a combination of these and many other factors. I will teach you about true nutrition and what your mind and body need to change for the long haul, but it does take commitment and patience from you for the next 21 days and beyond. Commit to modifying your habits without extremes and I promise you will feel so much better with time. Instead of starting and stopping a set of strict rules over and over again, you will start to solidify healthier habits and a more realistic way of thinking. Although I don't subscribe to a dieting mentality, I do find it helpful to use tools like implementing some structure, maintaining accountability, and following the guidelines of science-backed nutrition so that your metabolism works most efficiently and your body is naturally able to let go of excess weight. You want everything right now but your new mind and body cannot get delivered overnight. Your body is too smart to change that quickly and it does take work. Years, decades, or a lifetime of habits won't change overnight. But the more consistent you are, the more quickly you will see and feel results.

SET YOUR INTENTION

How often do you wake up and criticize yourself right away? It usually has something to do with how "badly" you ate yesterday, what part of your body you don't like, or just a general feeling of gloom that there is no solution and you will never be able to change. You feel like you have failed so many times in the quest for that magic pill to feel happy and healthy. Here we go again.

This might sound silly but that magic does exist and it's not a medication, a trendy diet, or a supplement: It's you. You have the power within you but maybe you haven't been given the proper nutritional advice or you haven't been in the right mind-set yet. There's an overwhelming amount of conflicting, confusing advice out there, so it's not your fault if you've had some missteps.

But the train to Negative Town ends now. Wake up each morning, pour yourself a big glass of water before food or coffee, and say aloud or write down at least one positive thing about yourself. Set an intention for realistic baby steps every day and commit to patience and imperfection in this process. It takes time to change that hardwired, stubborn brain of yours but I'm here to give you the factual nutrition lowdown and help you through it.

BECOME YOUR OWN BEST FRIEND

When it comes to losing weight, you tend to become your own worst enemy. Once you start to feel better and make progress, you tell yourself that you "deserve" rewards, which are usually in the form of food, and then you self-sabotage and can't bounce back. Once you veer from a "plan," that loss-of-control switch flips in your brain and one treat leads to another and another, and suddenly, you're in a more defeated place than where you began. Think of tempering your thoughts and slowly adjusting them, instead of flipping the switch on and off. I know you want a solid answer when it comes to your diet, something exact to swallow or follow but you know that never lasts. Nutrition is not black and white and you are not a robot, so give yourself a break.

Rather than considering weight loss as cut-and-dried, think of it as a very imperfect process of figuring yourself out. Practice including all foods in your diet, even ones that were off-limits in your mind before. You will learn to balance the treats that you love and that are totally worth indulging in, like a warm chocolate chip cookie (vs. that packaged cookie that can sit on the grocery shelf for years), with plenty of healthy, fresh options. In order to maintain a healthy and happy way of life that becomes second nature, it is important to learn how to live in the best of both worlds when it comes to your diet so you never feel deprived. If you continue to restrict and deprive yourself of certain foods you enjoy, then you will end up overdoing it when those cookies are in front of you again.

When you start to make progress, push even harder through those sabotaging thoughts. Talking yourself into something can go both ways and your brain is your most powerful tool. We talk to ourselves all day long and food is usually front and center, so instead of the same old thoughts, replace them with different, more empowering outcomes. Rather than rewarding yourself with food, try doing something that makes you happy, like reading your favorite trashy magazine, catching up on a TV series, or getting a manicure and mini massage. After the initial 21 days in this book and a well-deserved pat on the back, maybe you even spring for a blender upgrade so you can make even more recipes!

Your brain will eventually begin to believe you, even if you really don't believe yourself right now, and you will make healthier decisions. You will start to change your thought process and become your own best friend.

LIVE IN THE NOW AND DON'T OVERCOMPLICATE ANYTHING

Stop living in the past or looking to the future, and instead focus on right now. Your past can hold you back from moving forward but forget what struggles you've been through and just remember that it all happened to bring you right here, right now. Take each situation as it comes. It's easy to read this, get psyched up, and feel motivated that this time you are going to succeed. But when situations come up and you are in the moment, you may struggle to make the healthy decisions you were so excited to make. These situations can happen many times a day, so try imagining how you'll feel afterward based on which decision you make. Will eating a few extra cookies at the company holiday party make you feel good and happy afterward, because they're special and you'll have FOMO if you don't eat them? Or have you had them tons of times, they're unnecessary extras, and you'll feel too full after? If you start relaxing and listening to your body and what it needs instead of overthinking every piece of diet advice you've ever heard, you will move into a better place and your health and weight will benefit.

GET YOUR KITCHEN RIGHT

Now that we've covered getting your noggin prepared to create healthier habits, let's get your kitchen equipped to start blending away. Although there is a wide variety of recipes in this book, don't overcomplicate the smoothie-making process. Take these recipes, use them as a guide for ideas, and modify them based on what ingredients you currently have and what appeals to you most.

ESSENTIAL SMOOTHIE COMPONENTS

Every smoothie is intended to act as a meal or snack and should contain some basic nutrition components to fill you up and keep you satisfied. These ingredients include fruits; veggies; liquids such as different milks, water, or coffee; and a protein option such as nuts or seeds, nut or seed butters, different yogurts, or protein powders.

Vegetables

A plant-based diet may appear to be all the rage now, but the truth is, dietitians have always recommended a diet full of veggies. Although you may not struggle as much to get sweet fruits into your diet, your veggie intake always needs a boost and there is no easier way to sneak veggies into your diet than in a smoothie. A veggie will add tons of different vitamins, minerals, and fiber to your shake and boost the antioxidant factor even more. The choice is yours when deciding between fresh and frozen veggies but I'll let you in on a secret: Frozen veggies can actually be even more nutritious than fresh because they're frozen at the peak of freshness! The travel and transport time from farm to table is likely many days, so by the time you actually eat fresh veggies, they will have lost some nutrients. Frozen veggies also last for a long time in the freezer, unlike the fresh ones, so it's a smart idea to keep a couple bags of cauliflower rice, sweet potatoes, carrots, and greens in your freezer so you always have them in a pinch and there's no washing or cutting needed. Frozen cauliflower is great for thickening smoothies and canned pumpkin puree can make a tasty and nutritious addition as well. Shortcuts are the name of the game!

Fruits

Just as with veggies, I recommend buying bags of frozen fruit because of the preserved nutrient content, greater availability, and ease in prep, as they're ready-to-go, and because frozen fruit provides the frosty cold texture in a smoothie without the use of ice cubes. My top frozen picks for smoothies are berries for their high fiber and low sugar content; cherries for their rich color, sweetness, and high antioxidant content; mango for its sweet flavor and boost of vitamin C; and other exotic fruits that are ready to use, such as pineapple, coconut, acai, and cranberries, for their high fiber, vitamin, and mineral content.

Frozen fruits are available all year long and you'll be able to incorporate more exotic, nutrient-rich fruits into your diet than you would normally eat. When do you eat cranberries other than on a holiday or in the dried, high-sugar version? I even discovered frozen avocado chunks in the local supermarket recently and it made my day.

Last but not least, bananas are the most versatile fruit option in any ingredient combo because they provide just the right hit of sweetness that will make even the greenest smoothie taste good. Plus, you can buy bananas anywhere, they're uber economical, and you can peel them and freeze them in an airtight bag for future speedy use.

Liquids

Once you choose your fruits and veggies, you'll need a liquid vehicle to blend it all up. The variety of different milks on the market these days is astounding! From dairy to dairy-free alternatives like oat, coconut, pea protein, hemp, macadamia, and walnut, your choices are endless— depending on your specific dietary needs or preferences. Good old dairy, soy, or almond milk work great, too, and are available everywhere, so keep it simple and use any variety you prefer. I recommend unsweetened milks if available, so make sure you look at the label closely and choose ones without added sugar. If you like juice, use it to add a splash of sweetness and flavor instead of as the main liquid option because it has a much higher sugar content than most milks. Water is also always an option but most milks provide some added protein and nutrients to your smoothie. Some recipes include coffee and tea as a liquid option, too, so the hardest choice will be deciding which smoothie to make first.

Nuts, Nut Butters, and Proteins

In addition to the carbohydrate base of fruits and veggies, it is important to add a source of protein that will help slow down digestion, keep your blood sugar stable, and round out your smoothie into a complete meal or snack. Use quality protein options such as unsweetened plain regular or Greek yogurt; nondairy plant-based yogurts like coconut, almond, and even pili/plantain yogurt (called Lavva); unsweetened plain protein powders such as whey, pea, or hemp; and nut and seed butters like almond, peanut, and cashew nut butter and sunflower, pumpkin, and watermelon seed butter. Not only do they provide filling protein and nutrition but they also fit perfectly into the mostly sweet flavor and texture profiles of smoothies. My top super-seed picks for an extra nutrition boost in a smoothie are chia, hemp, and flaxseed, and you can even buy combo bags now that contain all three.

THE BLENDER

There is no smoothie-making magic without a blender. If you don't have a decent one in the house yet, I would recommend searching online for blender price comparisons and finding a great one on sale. Although I did invest in a Vitamix years ago and tested all the recipes in this book with it, you do not have to spend hundreds of dollars on a top-of-the-line brand. A Vitamix or Blendtec can do much more than make a simple smoothie and they are not necessary for you to "slim down with smoothies," but they are hands-down the most powerful blenders on the market and give smoothies an excellent creamy texture no matter what the ingredients happen to be. These machines incorporate veggies so well that even picky kids won't detect them. I can't say the same for a low-wattage machine. Recently, however, the variety of excellent blenders on the market has increased and prices have decreased, so there is no better time than now to find your shiny new smoothie-making friend.

Wattage

Power is everything when it comes to creating a smooth, creamy texture, especially when there are more fibrous fruits and veggies and tougher solid ingredients like seeds and nuts. When you're looking for a blender, go for the higher wattage, with at least 600 watts of power, so no ingredient stands a chance of being left out of the friendly mix. The more power, the better, so make wattage a priority when you're ready to buy.

Stainless Steel Blades

Most blenders on the market these days have stainless steel blades but when you're doing your research, just make sure of it. Stainless blades are the sharpest and most powerful type, so in addition to the wattage of the machine, the actual blades are also important for creating the best smoothie texture.

Size

Size matters but it depends on your individual smoothie-making needs. If you're making more than two servings of a smoothie at a time, make sure the capacity of the container is large enough to accommodate all of your ingredients. The smoothies in this book serve two, so a smaller "bullet" machine is more than enough and will take up less space on your counter.

Cleanup

A Vitamix container is not dishwasher safe, but a quick rinse is all it needs for the next batch. A dishwasher-safe machine would be a bonus though, because whatever affords you less cleanup and makes your life easier in any way is worth considering when you're in the market for a blender.

Speed Settings

If you have the ability to control the speed of blending, this feature is a bonus because you can adjust it based on the textures of the ingredients. By having the option to turn a dial up or down, you have more control over the final outcome of the smoothie texture and can incorporate more resilient ingredients that a single-speed blender may not be able to handle as well.

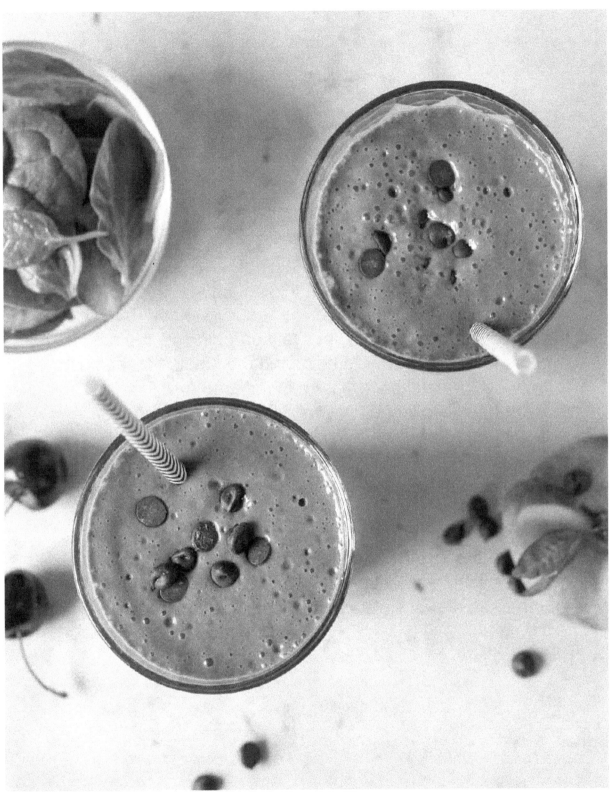

Dark Chocolate Star

Chapter Two
PREPPING FOR THE PLAN

I CAN'T BEGIN TO TELL YOU how pumped I am that you're ready to make the commitment to slim down with smoothies! Now that you're armed with all the tools you need to get on the smoothie-making train, let's talk prepping for the next 21 days so this plan is easy-breezy and the habits you begin to form will become second nature in the long run. Just remember, this is a healthy way of eating where you will actually feel satisfied and enjoy what you're eating and drinking instead of following another restrictive diet. The addition of nutritious and filling smoothies, coupled with my favorite solid meal and snack suggestions (while also teaching you the evidence-based reasons behind this way of eating), is the key to clearing up your confusion and struggles with food. Let's ditch the diet mentality and do this together the responsible way.

LOADING THE BLENDER

I love smoothies for many reasons, but the fact that there is no exact science behind the loading and blending process is at the top of my list. No one has time to worry about precise amounts of anything when it comes to preparing and eating food, but throwing ingredients into one container, pushing a button, and ending up with a tasty, healthy treat is doable for anyone. With a powerful blender, I have found that you can load the ingredients in any order and the blades will easily mix them up. However, with a standard blender, follow this order to ensure a perfectly blended shake:

LIQUID

You cannot make a smoothie without liquid, so start here and pour it in first. This is the one ingredient that is required for blending up all the others. Based on the other specific ingredients and whether there are frozen or solid components, like fruits and ice cubes or tough seeds or nuts, you can easily adjust the amount of liquid or just add extra water to get the blades moving and produce the desired consistency.

PROTEIN BASE

After adding the liquid, choose your protein(s) to keep your blood sugar and hunger levels stable and transform your smoothie into a complete meal. A powerful blender can easily crush whole nuts and seeds but you can use creamy or crunchy butters as a good protein and healthy fat addition, too.

FRUITS AND VEGETABLES

After you layer the initial liquid and proteins into the container, pick your produce. Use any variety of fresh and frozen fruits and veggies and add them on top of the protein and liquid tiers to create the main flavor and texture of the smoothie. Depending on which recipe and flavor combo you choose, you can decide whether fresh or frozen options make more sense to create the consistency and chill factor you want in your drink.

You can add extras at any point in the blending process but you can also just think of this final step as the cherry on top. Add a sprinkle of additional spices, powders, extracts, and seeds at the end to add some extra flavor and pizzazz to your already-nutritious smoothie. After you pour the smoothie into a glass, you can add a touch of chocolate chips, oats, cinnamon, or additional sliced fruit right on top to enhance the presentation and taste. Who doesn't like a little extra excitement in their food? Experimenting with smoothies and eating healthier in general can also be fun, which is an important part of the process. Plus, good-looking meals enhance your eating experience and can make you feel even more satisfied with your choices.

EXTRA, EXTRA!

Your health will benefit from simply modifying your basic dietary habits, but let's explore the oodles of additions that can enhance the taste, texture, and nutrition of your recipes. Although these extras are not necessary for success on the plan, they can spice up and pack an additional nutrition punch into your diet, which is always a bonus.

- If you need more sustenance, like after a tough workout, add an extra scoop of protein powder, yogurt, or nut/seed butter.

- Spices like cinnamon, ginger, and nutmeg add sweetness and antioxidants without any sugar.
- Turmeric is a powerful antioxidant and bright yellow spice that you can add to specific smoothie recipes as well.
- Matcha (green tea powder) is another antioxidant superfood and provides a bitter flavor that balances out and tastes

delicious when combined with creamy and sweet ingredients. Matcha and chai spice blends are included in some of the recipes, but make sure to buy the unsweetened brands.

- Pure vanilla, almond, and mint extracts can add a touch of flavor without added sugar.
- There are also a variety of superfood powders on the market now, like green, red, and blue powders, which add vitamins, minerals, polyphenols, phytonutrients, and antioxidants. Essentially, they're nutrient compounds found in certain plant foods that can help the body defend itself from developing cardiovascular diseases and cancers and may assist with overall health, like digestion, immunity, and inflammation.

These superfood additions can help your body protect itself but only if you are already living a generally healthy lifestyle to begin with. So, if you want to experiment with some extras, keep it simple and remember to keep your focus on eating real foods first.

OPTIONAL NUTRITIONAL BOOSTERS

PROTEIN POWDERS	SPICES/ HERBS/ EXTRACTS	SEEDS	NUT BUTTERS	SUPERFOOD POWDERS	PURÉES	GRAINS/ BEANS/ SOY
Plain collagen powder	Cayenne	Basil	Almond	Bee pollen	Pumpkin	Black beans
Plain hemp protein	Cilantro	Chia	Cashew	Cacao	Sweet potato	Oats
Plain pea protein	Cinnamon	Flax	Macadamia nut	Coffee flour		Tofu
Plain whey protein	Ginger	Hemp	Peanut	Espresso		White beans

Mint	Sunflower seed	Pumpkin	Greens
Nutmeg	Sunflower seed		Maca
Parsley	Walnut		Matcha
Pure almond extract	Watermelon seed		Prebiotic and probiotic
Pure vanilla extract			Spirulina
Turmeric			

BUILDING A HEALTHY WHOLE-FOOD MEAL

The majority of your diet both during and after the 21 days should include meals full of real, fresh foods, with one or two smoothies per day depending on your preference. Envision your day as including three meals and one or two snacks, with a smoothie as either a meal or a snack replacement, for a total of four or five mealtimes per day. Meals should include a serving of carbohydrates, a protein and fat source, and as many veggies as you can pack into your day. Veggies add volume to meals and are the key to being able to both visually and physically eat more while consuming fewer calories. Just imagine your plate as one-quarter protein, such as grilled chicken; one-quarter carbs/starch, such as a small baked potato; and half veggies, such as a big raw salad or roasted mixed veggies.

There are no concrete rules when it comes to mealtimes, as individual schedules differ greatly, but your meals should generally keep you full for around three hours. If they don't, that's a sign to add more food. Feel free to have your smoothie or two for any meal or snack at any time of day.

The most common cause of weight gain that I see is a lack of adequate food intake during the day. When you're busy and running around, you're more distracted and just don't notice hunger as much. The typical scenario is a blood sugar crash in the late afternoon or evening, so when you get home, the food floodgates open wide. You raid the kitchen with little to no control and can't stop eating until bedtime because your body is making up for lost calories and more. When the majority of calories are consumed later in the day and at night, your body cannot use the energy as efficiently. You just don't need as much fuel later when you're usually home relaxing and going to bed shortly thereafter.

Quick meal ideas are my main jam, so let's discuss what a meal should look like so you can picture what to include with each one.

LEAN PROTEIN

Imagine one-quarter of your plate as a serving of grilled, broiled, lightly sautéed, or roasted protein, such as chicken, turkey, fish, shellfish, lean beef, pork, eggs, egg whites, nuts, seeds, tofu, tempeh, or veggie burger; or a serving of dairy, such as cheese or yogurt.

Generally, for women, 4 to 6 ounces of protein with each meal (a portion about the size of 1½ to 2 decks of playing cards) is adequate. Examples include 2 eggs, 20 to 25 nuts, ⅛ cup of seeds, or 1 cup of milk or yogurt.

For men, 6 to 8 ounces is appropriate (a portion about the size of 2 to 3 decks of playing cards). Examples include 3 eggs, 30 to 40 nuts, ¼ cup of seeds, or 1½ cups of milk or yogurt.

VEGGIES

When it comes to veggies, as long as they're prepared with few or no sauces and extra oils, the sky is the limit. If there is any way at all to add veggies to your food, remember that more is always better because they're the best caloric bang for your buck. They provide the most filling nutrition and volume for the least amount of calories. We are not gaining weight from eating too many veggies, so pile them on! Anything goes, from raw salads to roasted broccoli to veggie soups. Munch on them between meals and with snacks, too. If you're going to mindlessly munch, skip the chips and stick with veggies.

HEART-HEALTHY FATS

Most of the previously listed proteins contain fat naturally but feel free to add extra fat if needed. Healthy fat options include ¼ to ½ of a small avocado; 1 to 2 tablespoons of olive, avocado, or coconut oil or a healthy salad dressing on your veggies; or a sprinkle of additional seeds or nuts. A serving of extra fat in your meals can be the missing piece of the puzzle to keep you consistently satisfied with your healthy choices and curb your sugar cravings.

NUTRITIOUS CARBS

Contrary to what you may have heard, carbohydrates are a very important part of your diet for sustainable, healthy weight loss. They should provide about half of the calories in your diet, as they are your brain's main source of fuel. However, we tend to overeat them because we are addicted to the processed versions like candy, cookies, or chips, or the super-starchy ones like bagels, baked goods, and pastas. I could write a book on carbs alone, but in a nutshell, there are two very different categories of carbs: Naked carbs are the ones without a label that grow outside, like fruit, and are your most nutritious sources. Processed carbs come in bags and boxes and can last for years on a grocery store shelf.

Choose the most nutritious, fiber-rich sources, such as fresh fruit, unprocessed sprouted bread and wraps (like Food for Life), whole-wheat bakery bread, whole-food crackers (like Mary's Gone Crackers), potatoes, brown rice, pasta, quinoa, beans, lentils, corn, and oats, and stick to one to two servings per meal. A standard serving of carbohydrates is about 15 grams, which equates to 1 thin slice of bread; ½ cup of cooked grains, rice, beans, or pasta; ½ cup of uncooked oats; 1 small piece of fruit; or 1 cup of fruit.

Check the ingredients first on any packaged food to make sure that you can understand the words and that it includes mostly real ingredients without fillers and added sugar. The majority of food on a shelf is processed and junky, so don't believe the claims on the box. The ingredients will give you the information you need to become your own food detective with time. Then check the label for the serving size and carbohydrate content to figure out what a portion looks like, so you are able to stick with one to two servings per meal.

SERVING SIZES FOR COMMON FOODS

It can be helpful—and eye-opening—to be aware of the portions you eat. Here are some serving size guidelines to follow:

EQUIVALENT		FOOD	CALORIES
Fist	¾ cup	Rice	150
		Pasta	150
		Potatoes	150
Palm	4 ounces	Lean meat	160
		Fish	160
		Poultry	160
Handful	1 ounce	Nuts	170
		Raisins	85
Thumb	1 ounce	Peanut butter	170
		Hard cheese	100

WHAT TO EXPECT

This new way of eating is going to change your health, as long as you are patient and consistent. Lasting change takes adjustment but just imagine how great you will feel after implementing a healthier way of living!

During the process of modifying your dietary habits and overall lifestyle, you can expect some changes in the beginning but don't be alarmed. These symptoms are your body's way of naturally detoxing and making room for a healthier you. Here is what you can expect as you transform your habits over the next few weeks and beyond.

IN THE SHORT RUN . . .

You May Crave Sugar

Whenever you begin to wean yourself off processed food and added sugar, you can expect withdrawal symptoms, and one of them is craving the sugar that your body has become so used to having. It may take a few days for the cravings to subside, but stay strong and focus on natural sources of sugar like the fruit in your smoothies.

You May Get Headaches

The withdrawal symptoms of less added sugar and possibly less caffeine—I encourage you to eat more during the day instead of just drinking coffee for energy—can result in headaches and irritability. Rest assured, these headaches will quickly pass and your natural energy levels will skyrocket.

Your Bowel Movements May Change

One of the first signs you will notice when you begin to change your diet is more consistent bowel movements, which means your body is working much better! A diet higher in real, high-fiber foods like fruits, veggies, and whole grains, coupled with drinking more water to lubricate this addition of fibrous material in your GI tract, almost always improves the quality and consistency of your pooping habits. That, in turn, can alleviate chronic constipation and assist with weight loss. I love to hear a client tell me they are pooping more frequently and are less bloated now. Healthier habits lead to a healthier GI tract, which is your body's center of immunity.

You May Be Urinating More

When you include more water-rich fruits and veggies in your diet and hydrate more in general, you may notice more frequent trips to the bathroom. Just as your bowel movements will improve, your increased need to pee indicates that your body is naturally self-detoxifying. When your urine becomes clear throughout the day, you can pat yourself on the back that you're doing a better job of hydrating.

Your Hunger Levels Will Stabilize, Especially at Night

When you properly fuel your body throughout the day instead of skipping meals and skimping on carbs, you will find your blood sugar and hunger levels are more stable, and you will not become ravenous later in the day. Now that you are eating every few hours and including enough carbs, protein, and fat in your meals, you will not be as hungry, and your dinners can be lighter. You will begin to wake up hungry in the morning, which is a great sign.

IN THE LONG RUN . . .

You Will Sleep Better

One of the most noteworthy changes you will experience when you adjust your diet is the shift in your sleeping patterns. Consistent positive dietary changes will promote quality sleep. Balanced meals throughout the day and a lighter meal at night will lead to better digestion, with less incidence of acid reflux, and a more well-rested night. When your sleep improves, the hunger hormones ghrelin and leptin are in check, which will then help control hunger cues and cravings and aid in weight loss.

You Will Have More Energy

If you don't fuel a car when it's running on empty or keep up with oil changes, it will begin to break down. The same is true of your body.

When you fuel it properly, your energy levels stabilize and those slumps will begin to dissipate. As you couple this with the likelihood of more quality sleep, you will bounce out of bed more easily, and your performance at work, during workouts, and in everyday life will be boosted. You may even have more patience with your kids! You may not notice it at first but you will start feeling better without the need for sugary pick-me-ups and caffeinated beverages throughout the day because you are now fueling with nutritious food.

Your Appearance Will Improve

There is no better remedy for improving your appearance than eating a nutrient-rich diet and hydrating well. This healthy way of eating will transform you from the inside out and will likely improve your hair, skin, and nails. Most important, you will feel empowered by food and your confidence will soar, so you will naturally be glowing, too. No facials or Botox needed!

You Will Feel Lighter and Less Bloated

Not only will you feel mentally lighter but your body will lose excess water weight from replacing processed foods with more water, fiber, and nutrient-dense options. Your body has a natural detox system—the kidneys and liver—and is able to get rid of waste and fluid efficiently, especially when your habits are swapped for healthier ones. Plus, when hormones are better regulated by eating well, hydrating, moving more, etc., your body releases excess retained water, and that icky feeling of bloat resolves.

Your Weight Will Naturally Move

By the end of the initial 21 days, not only will your mind and body feel much lighter and happier, but your weight should gradually move in a healthier direction. When you eat balanced meals in appropriate portions throughout the day, your weight will naturally adjust. So instead of living by that number on the scale, which will fluctuate on an hourly basis for a million different reasons, focus on changing your habits with patience and the weight loss will come with time.

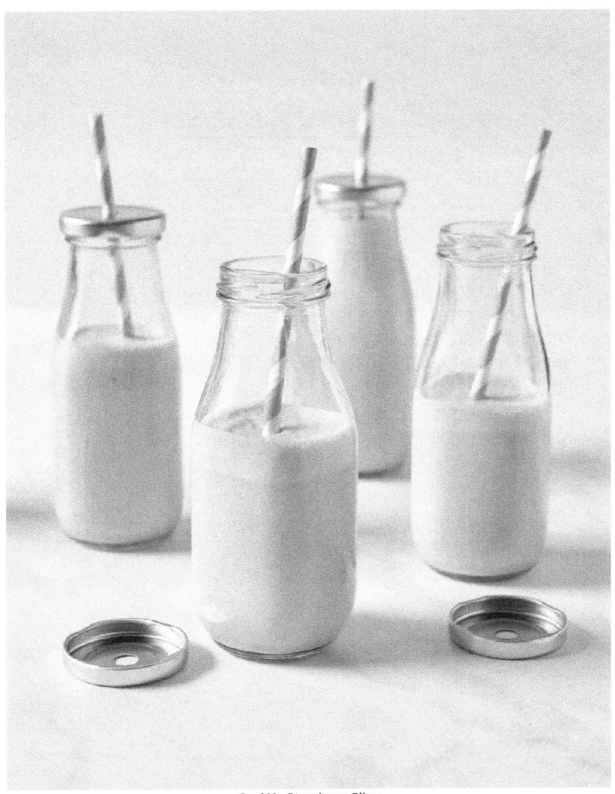

Caul Me Strawberry Slims

Chapter Three
PARAMETERS OF
THE PLAN

I BET YOU CAN'T CONTAIN YOUR EXCITEMENT and want to get right to it, so I won't make you wait any longer. Your new way of eating should be simple, realistic, and straightforward, and if it's not, I give you permission to pour a smoothie over my head. Remember that allowing yourself time to adjust to new habits is imperative for lasting change. Smiling and enjoying your meals is not mandatory but highly recommended in my nutrition playbook (and in this book).

5 SIMPLE GUIDELINES

Think of healthy eating as a set of general guidelines that enables you to have both structure for weight loss and flexibility to adjust to any life situation. This thought process is essential to ending the short-lived diet mentality that you've been through countless times in the past. In this plan, you can choose whether you prefer to drink a smoothie one or two times a day, and then fill in the other meals and snacks with whole foods.

1. Plan your day so that you will be eating every 3 to 4 hours, which is the general time frame in which your body has digested the last meal and needs to refuel. Adjust your mealtimes based on your schedule for that particular day.

2. Drink a smoothie or have a whole-foods breakfast.

3. Drink a smoothie or have a whole-foods lunch.

4. Eat one or two recommended snacks throughout the day. Mix and match a carbohydrate and protein option from the following list. Typically, I suggest a snack between breakfast and lunch if needed, but don't skip the afternoon snack between lunch and dinner, so that your dinner meal is as light as possible. This is a key factor in promoting weight loss.

Snack Pick Guide: Carb + Protein/Fat + Veggies

- ♦ **The Elvis:** Banana (carb) + 1 tablespoon of natural nut or seed butter such as peanut, almond, or sunflower seed butter (protein/fat)
- ♦ **Fruit + Nuts:** Apple (carb) + 25 nuts or ⅛ cup of seeds (protein/fat)
- ♦ **Choco Nut:** 2 small squares (½ ounce) of 70 percent or more dark chocolate (carb) + 25 nuts or ⅛ cup of seeds (protein/fat)
- ♦ **Yogurt Parfait:** 1 cup of berries (carb) + 1 cup of plain 2 percent Greek yogurt (protein/fat)

- ♦ **Crax + Eggs:** 1 serving of whole-grain crackers such as Mary's Gone Crackers (carb) + 2 hardboiled eggs (protein/fat) with everything bagel seasoning (optional but amazing) + raw veggies
- ♦ **Fruit + Cheese:** 1 sliced pear (carb) + 1 or 2 string cheeses or other single-serving cheese option (protein/fat) + raw veggies
- ♦ **Crudité:** 1 serving of whole-grain crackers (carb) + 2 tablespoons of hummus or guacamole (or a single-serving pack) (protein/fat) + raw veggies
- ♦ **Avocado Toast:** 1 thin slice of grainy toast (carb) + ½ mashed avocado (fat) + 1 slice of cheese or 1 egg (protein/fat) + raw veggies

Feel free to add veggies or ¼ of a sliced avocado to any snack option listed here. The more veggies, the better!

5. Eat a light but well-balanced dinner with a serving of protein, lots of raw or cooked veggies, and an optional serving of carbohydrates (such as a small baked potato).

One of the best things you can do for weight loss is to refrain from continuing to eat after dinner and give yourself 10 to 12 hours of digestive rest. "Close down" the kitchen, have a cup of tea to relax, and brush and floss to help signal your body that it's time to hit the sack soon!

10 TIPS FOR SLIM DOWN SUCCESS

I love a good top 10 list, so let me give you the 411 on how to successfully slim down the smart and sensible way.

1. **Legit commit.** For the best shot at scoring permanent success, there is nothing more essential than mentally

committing to a process, believing in yourself, and maintaining extra patience while you go through the ups and downs. Without this realistic mind-set from the get-go, you will continue to go in endless circles of dieting defeat.

2. **Feed the furnace.** Eat enough (including carbohydrates) throughout the day and taper off your food intake toward the end of the day. If you fuel your body adequately during the day, your hangry nighttime nemesis will hit the road and you will not miss him one bit. You will notice that afternoon energy slumps and cravings fade and your dinner meals will become lighter and commensurate with your intake during the day.

3. **Chug water like a champ.** Don't tell me you don't like water because I've heard that one before. Nutrition fun facts are my favorite, and the fact is, you are mostly made up of water (55 to 65 percent on average) and every function in your body requires water, so practice hydrating more and make water your new BFF. Aim for 2 to 3 liters a day, or 64 to 96 ounces.

4. **Optimize your zzzz's.** Evaluate your sleep habits and make it a priority to get 7 to 8 hours a night. I know how hard this is for most of us, because we all lead busy lives, but sleep is a time when your body heals and repairs itself and resets all of your hormones that will spill over into the way you feel— and the food choices you make—the next day. Good night, sleep tight.

5. **Address the stress.** We all have stress but there are ways to help minimize it so that it doesn't wreak havoc on your health. Journaling your thoughts, getting a massage, going to yoga, listening to music, walking, or anything that relaxes you is a good idea. Just stopping and taking a few deep breaths can make a world of difference. I know it sounds silly, but try it and you may be pleasantly surprised at how the little things add up to a calmer you.

6. **Volumize veggies.** Add veggies anywhere you can for volume. They are by far the best caloric bang for your buck for the most nutrition. The more you fill your plates and bowls with them, the more you can eat and the less you will take in naturally.

7. **Check yourself before you wreck yourself.** I will provide you with all the tools you need for success but the truth is, accountability is more than half the battle. Hold yourself accountable and stay consistent with your new habits by keeping a food journal, writing notes in your phone, or finding a coach or friend to report to on a weekly basis. Do what will realistically work for you.

8. **Move more.** Don't go from zero to 60 with exercise; simply do anything more than you're doing now. Walking up the stairs instead of using the elevator and parking farther away from the store both count as "more." When you're ready, adding weight training and resistance exercises can increase your muscle mass and metabolism and create a leaner, meaner you.

9. **Slow down to slim down.** Stop rushing around, walking, or standing while you eat. I bet you don't even put your fork down during an entire meal at times, and you are likely distracted by something with a screen. We eat quickly and don't pay attention during mealtimes, so our bodies fail to register what we just ate and we continue to eat after we've had enough. Sit at a table, put your utensils down, take sips of water between bites, and minimize distractions so you can enjoy and savor your food.

10. **Cut the crap.** I'm talking processed foods and added sugars. Stick with real, unprocessed foods as outlined in this plan and limit the sweets like candy, cookies, ice cream, and other packaged stuff that loads added sugar into your diet and makes it harder to stick to healthy habits. The sugar monster is real and the less you give in to its luring ways, the

better.

FIGHT FATIGUE AND PREVENT GETTING HANGRY

Most restrictive diets can sap you of all your energy because you're not fueling yourself properly. You may feel tired, cranky, and irritable, or what I refer to as classic "hangry," simply because you are hungry and angry from a lack of food. This sluggish feeling is likely a result of low blood sugar and is often accompanied by a headache. If you are experiencing hangry symptoms, please stop, drop, and eat more food because no one will want to be around you, including yourself! If you're experiencing fatigue, evaluate your meals for adequacy, and make sure you're getting enough water and sleep as well. Listen to your body and add more sustenance to your meals and snacks so you are satisfied. Add extra-satiating protein and fats, such as avocado, an egg, chicken or turkey, olive oil, or nuts and seeds. When you begin changing your habits for the better and eating enough food like in the sample plan in this book (and adding more as needed), you should actually feel quite the opposite. You will have more energy to keep going and going and going . . . You get the point.

IF YOU HAVE A SETBACK

I hope you know by now that I am going to be 100 percent honest with you when it comes to realistic weight loss and what it's going to take for you to meet your goals and maintain them. The road is never completely smooth, even when you are drinking smoothies. You have to expect setbacks because they will absolutely happen but the best thing you can do is to keep moving. Put the gloves away, because there's no point in beating yourself up. Instead, think of all the positive changes you have already made. You have the control to swap every negative thought for a positive one, and believe me, this new mind-set feels so much better. It's much easier to give up and revert to old habits when you've veered from a set plan, but I can't stress enough that you will never be able to stick to exact rules and regulations for more than a finite amount of time. Plus, that's just boring anyway. Look at the big picture and imagine what it would be like if this time was different. What if this time, you gave yourself a break and changed the right way, by expecting imperfection and allowing your mind and body the opportunity to finally learn and adjust without fixed limits? Think of all the time you will actually end up saving because instead of having to follow endless rules again and again without success, you will have changed for good.

MOVE THAT BODY!

We already touched on this briefly but it's time to get your tush moving! Although dietary changes are the most effective way to lose weight and improve your overall health, there are overwhelming benefits to leading an active lifestyle. First of all, there is nothing like a good workout to keep your motivation sky-high for eating well and taking care of yourself. It's no wonder most gyms have smoothie bars. A good sweat and a refreshing smoothie afterward go hand in hand. The best natural high and boost of self-confidence come after you move your body, so think of a simple way you can incorporate more movement into your schedule.

Start really small and be realistic: What will you actually do and when? Anything goes, even just walking for 20 to 30 minutes at least 3 days a week. Schedule walks in your calendar just like you would any appointment so that you actually stick to it. The hardest part is getting started but when you do, you may find yourself walking longer than you expected. With time, your endurance will improve and you can add weight resistance exercises like push-ups, sit-ups, and more (even with arm and leg weights) to boost your metabolism and assist with weight loss. Building lean muscle mass is one of the most effective ways to change your body composition and help maintain your weight when you get to a happy place. Plus, for those of you who really love to eat, like me, staying in good shape helps you get away with indulging a bit more (but shhh, that's our little secret).

AFTER THE PLAN

The plan in this book is just a starting point so don't panic when it "ends." Healthy eating is a continuous choice and takes effort to get to a point where your new habits just become your normal life. I encourage you to use these healthy-eating guidelines paired with nutritious smoothies to promote lifelong health.

HOW TO MAINTAIN YOUR WEIGHT LOSS

The beauty of ditching diets and doing this the right way is that if you are patient and your body changes slowly enough, you won't just suddenly gain weight back. When your body gets used to you at a new weight, you are able to maintain it plus or minus a few fluctuating pounds. If you constantly lose and gain 10-, 15-, or 20-plus pounds, this is a direct result of going on a restrictive diet, losing water weight, and then hitting a point where your body won't stand for it anymore (to protect you), and now you're eating everything in sight. Sound familiar? Remember, your body is too smart and won't let you get away with being super restrictive for too long.

Weight maintenance is also the stage where I want to reiterate the benefits of consistent exercise. Focus on building muscle mass and continue to get into better shape and your body will hover in a healthy place without ever having to go from one extreme of eating to another like you have in the past. There is really only one way of eating healthy despite all you've heard, so the guidelines you have learned won't suddenly change like they do on circulating fad diets. You can feel confident that you're eating healthy and your body will reward you by maintaining a healthy weight without so much struggle. Thank you, amazing body!

WHAT IF I DIDN'T LOSE WEIGHT?

Here's the thing: There's no timeline when it comes to weight loss. Give yourself a break if the scale isn't moving yet. Most people give up because they rely on a fickle scale and let an unreliable number dictate their existence. It's like all those weeks of effort and positive changes are immediately erased in the flash of a number. Throw that two-faced scale out the window if you must because you're smarter than that! I can assure you that by focusing on mostly real, whole foods and the other lifestyle recommendations I discuss in this book, you will eventually meet your goals. Think of even the smallest changes you have made and how much lighter you may feel in your mind and in the way your clothes fit. Most of all, remember that your health is changing on the inside and adding years to your life even if that moody scale hasn't accurately reflected this yet.

NEXT STEPS

Your quest for wellness has just begun and although this plan may feel like a jumping-off point, it is also just a healthy, responsible eating plan that can be used as a lifelong guide, because you know I do real-life, not-crazy diets. Take each new week as a chance to solidify your habits even further. New habits are like seeds that will eventually form roots, so be patient and let them grow with time. Keep adding to your progress with baby steps each week and remember that the path may be a little bumpy but it's so worth it! When the you-know-what hits the fan in life (which it always does), instead of taking several steps backward, this time you have the power to push forward and come out stronger and healthier.

MAKE ADJUSTMENTS

Unlike the smoothie recipes in this book, you don't come with directions. Please adjust any aspect of your particular lifestyle that isn't working well for you. There is really no right or wrong when it comes to staying on track with your health so think about what's working for you and what isn't. What tools are helping you stay accountable? What are you struggling with and what can you work on this week? With each week—even each day—comes a new opportunity to modify habits that will bring you closer to meeting your goals and feeling even more awesome.

SMOOTHIE TIPS

If you have ripe bananas, don't toss them! Instead, peel them and store them in a freezer-safe bag or container in the freezer for an easy smoothie addition. The same goes for any other fresh fruit, veggie, or herb. You can even cut them up and freeze them with a bit of water in an ice cube tray and use as needed.

Store leftover smoothies in the refrigerator in a container for up to three days. When you are ready to drink, you can pour the remainder back into the blender with ice to revive the texture.

Pour smoothies into a bowl and top with a sprinkle of fruit, granola, coconut, seeds, nuts, or other toppings to create a meal that you can eat with a spoon.

Pour leftover smoothies into ice-pop molds and place them in the freezer. When they freeze and are ready to eat, you have a tasty healthy treat for you and your family to enjoy later instead of relying on the packaged sugary options.

ABOUT THE RECIPES

The original recipes in this book are versions of smoothie recipes I have recommended throughout my career to assist people just like you with their health and weight-loss goals. They're fun, flavorful, and filled with tons of nourishing, satisfying, and easy-to-find whole-food ingredients. You can get as creative as you want but keep in mind that you can also keep it super simple and just rotate through a few of your favorites that have similar ingredients. Feel free to mix and match fruits and veggies, liquids, and proteins in amounts similar to those listed in the recipes, and the nutrient profiles won't drastically change. Adjust the contents to your liking and think of a smoothie as a big cold mess of goodness that you can't get wrong. That's the beauty of incorporating these blends into your diet: You can use them as guidelines for inspiration, but just like when setting health goals, it's a good idea to anticipate imperfection. As long as you're practicing healthier habits and being mindful of your food choices, you will feel and see a difference in your mind and body with time.

Although I used a variety of milks and protein additions to come up with 100 different smoothies (phew!), there is no need to buy more than one liquid and one protein, especially at first. My favorite staples that can be used in any of these recipes are good old plain Greek yogurt and unsweetened almond milk. If you ever need more liquid for blending, feel free to add more of the liquid in the recipe, or water always works, too.

I used 2 percent plain Greek yogurt in most of the recipes because of its high protein content and the creaminess factor it adds to the smoothies. Note that Greek and Icelandic yogurts yield the highest protein content in dairy yogurts, while the plant-based options are actually a poor source of protein. If you are able to tolerate dairy, I recommend using these plain yogurts first as your best protein option, because they have no added sugar and fillers. Although I usually use low-fat Greek yogurt for a tastier and more satisfying option than nonfat, I recommend choosing any fat percentage as long as the calorie difference is not significant. Smoothies are a great way to get the health benefits of eating yogurt without having to taste it in its plain, thick form.

To create a dairy-free version of any recipe, substitute some of my favorite healthy plant-based yogurts like plain coconut (Cocojune), pea protein (Ripple), almond milk (Kite Hill), or pili milk (Lavva), or use plain pea or hemp protein powder.

To create nut-free versions of any recipe, substitute dairy, coconut, oat, hemp, rice, or pea protein milk for almond milk. Substitute sunflower, pumpkin, or watermelon seed butter for almond butter and peanut butter.

Feel free to swap ingredients around to your liking but just make sure to include fruit, a protein, and a liquid. Veggie additions like kale, spinach, and other undetectable greens are always a welcome bonus. Most recipes use about 1 cup of fresh greens, but feel free to add more or less as desired.

These smoothies focus on using sources of natural sugar found in fruit instead of added sugar or artificial sweeteners, so you may find that they are not as sweet as you are used to. However, one of my goals with this book is to help you tackle that sugar addiction and wean you off that desire. Add a splash of natural sugar, like 100 percent fruit juice or a sweeter fruit like banana, mango, or pineapple, instead of adding honey, syrups, and sugars. Refrain from using any artificial sweeteners, as these processed chemicals are much sweeter than real sugar and can actually reinforce your need for sweets later in the day (because your tongue tastes sweet but no calories are absorbed, so your body will look for sweets elsewhere).

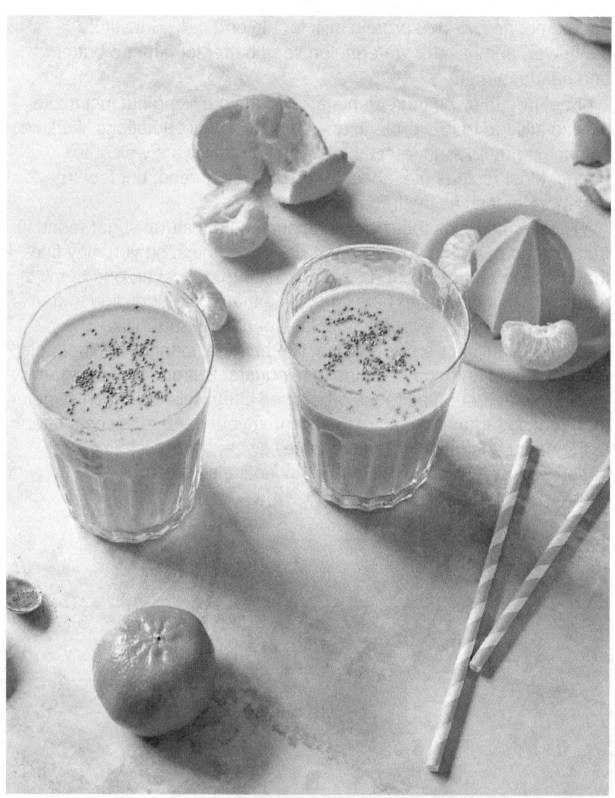

Classic Creamsicle

Chapter Four
21-DAY SMOOTHIE SLIM DOWN WEEK1

LET'S GET READY TO RUMBLE, smoothie-style! Welcome to your first week of suggested smoothie recipes. Remember to complement these blends with whole-food meals and snacks for this initial 21-day slim down. Think of these first three weeks as a starting point for trying different smoothie combos and you will discover which ones taste the best and also keep you the most satisfied. Stick with these picks and rotate as much or as little as you want but please keep your meal prep super easy so that you are consistent and begin to see as much change as possible. If you don't have some of the ingredients, it's okay to skip them as long as you have some sort of fruit paired with a liquid, such as milk or water, and a protein, such as yogurt, protein powder, or a nut/seed butter. The optional seeds and spices are recommended to round out the nutritional profile and flavor of the recipes. Head to the market to pick up some essentials and remember to keep in mind that having fun is part of the recipe for success!

WEEK 1 SHOPPING LIST

FRUITS AND VEGETABLES

- Avocado (1)
- Bananas (5)
- Spinach, baby (2 cups)

FROZEN

- Berries, mixed (1 cup)
- Blackberries (1 cup)
- Blueberries (2½ cups)
- Dragon fruit (1 [3.5-ounce] packet)
- Mangos (1 cup)
- Peaches (1 cup)
- Pineapple (1 cup)
- Strawberries (2 cups)

MILKS, NONDAIRY MILKS, AND YOGURTS

- Almond milk, unsweetened vanilla (1 [32-ounce] container)
- Coconut milk, unsweetened (refrigerated, not canned) (8 ounces)
- Dairy milk, nonfat or skim (1 [16-ounce] container)
- Yogurt, nonfat or low-fat plain Greek or Icelandic (1 [32-ounce] container)
- Yogurt, Siggi's low-fat or whole-milk vanilla (1 [24-ounce] container)

PANTRY

- Almond butter
- Cacao powder
- Chia seeds
- Chocolate hemp protein powder
- Cinnamon, ground
- Hemp seeds
- Oats, rolled

Big Blue

Anti-Inflammatory, Heart Health, Immune Boost

SERVES 2

Although this blend bursting with juicy, antioxidant- and fiber-rich berries may appear blue, there is nothing sad about it, so drink up and smile because healthy food makes you happy and pumps you full of energy, just like the big loving puppy named Blue that inspired this smoothie.

1 cup unsweetened vanilla almond milk

1 cup frozen blueberries

1 fresh or frozen banana

¾ cup plain low-fat Greek yogurt

1 tablespoon hemp seeds

1 tablespoon blue spirulina powder (optional)

In a blender, combine all the ingredients and blend until the desired consistency is achieved. Add more liquid as needed. Serve immediately.

Bonus Boost:

Berries are rich in fiber and when consumed as part of a high-fiber diet, they can help control blood sugar levels and maintain a healthy weight.

Per serving:

Calories: 245; Total fat: 6g; Sodium: 142mg; Cholesterol: 6mg; Total

carbs: 43g; Fiber: 8g; Sugar: 30g; Protein: 8g

HABIT TRACKER

Did you get 7 to 8 hours of sleep?   ☐Y ☐N

Did you drink 2 to 3 liters of water?   ☐Y ☐N

Did you exercise for at least 20 to 30 minutes?   ☐Y ☐N

Today's Big Win: ---

Goal(s) for Tomorrow: --

-

Emergency Chocolate

Heart Health

SERVES 2

Move over, sugar-filled cakes and cookies, because this nutritious chocolate smoothie takes care of your sweet tooth without the guilt when a chocolate emergency strikes. My favorite brand of protein powder for making this smoothie is Manitoba Harvest Chocolate Hemp Protein Powder.

1 cup unsweetened vanilla almond milk

1 cup frozen mixed berries

1 fresh or frozen banana

4 tablespoons chocolate hemp protein powder

1 tablespoon cacao powder

In a blender, combine all the ingredients and blend until the desired consistency is achieved. Add more liquid as needed. Serve immediately.

Bonus Boost:

This rich-tasting combo satisfies your cravings while also keeping your blood sugar and hunger stable due to the fiber from the fruit paired with plant-based hemp protein.

Per serving:

Calories: 206; Total fat: 2g; Sodium: 185mg; Cholesterol: 3mg; Total carbs: 31g; Fiber: 4g; Sugar: 12g; Protein: 19g

HABIT TRACKER

Did you get 7 to 8 hours of sleep?   ☐Y ☐N

Did you drink 2 to 3 liters of water?   ☐Y ☐N

Did you exercise for at least 20 to 30 minutes?   ☐Y ☐N

Today's Big Win: ---

Goal(s) for Tomorrow: --

-

The Bomb Pop

Heart Health

SERVES 2

Named for the classic summer red, white, and blue ice pop, this protein-rich smoothie that satisfies in any season will leave you feeling like da bomb. Exploding with fiber from the berries blended with seeds and yogurt, this combo will set off fireworks in your taste buds.

1 cup unsweetened vanilla almond milk

1 cup frozen blueberries

1 cup frozen strawberries

¾ cup plain low-fat Greek

yogurt 1 tablespoon chia seeds

In a blender, combine all the ingredients and blend until the desired consistency is achieved. Add more liquid as needed. Serve immediately.

Per serving:

Calories: 198; Total fat: 5g; Sodium: 144mg; Cholesterol: 6mg; Total carbs: 30g; Fiber: 7g; Sugar: 20g; Protein: 7g

HABIT TRACKER

Did you get 7 to 8 hours of sleep?	☐ Y	☐ N
Did you drink 2 to 3 liters of water?	☐ Y	☐ N
Did you exercise for at least 20 to 30 minutes?	☐ Y	☐ N

Today's Big Win: --

Goal(s) for Tomorrow: ---

Hot Pink Power

Anti-Inflammatory, Digestive Health, Heart Health

SERVES 2

This smoothie is too pink to be true. The hot pink color comes from a packet of frozen red dragon fruit, also known as pitaya, that you can find in most grocery stores. Dragon fruit is full of fiber, magnesium, and vitamin C, so blend it up with other ingredients and you'll feel pretty in hot pink in no time.

1 cup unsweetened coconut milk
1 cup frozen pineapple
¾ cup plain low-fat Greek yogurt
1 (3.5-ounce) packet frozen dragon fruit

In a blender, combine all the ingredients and blend until the desired consistency is achieved. Add more liquid as needed. Serve immediately.

Bonus Boost:

Lycopene, a cancer-protective antioxidant, is responsible for the dragon fruit's bright color.

Per serving:

Calories: 200; Total fat: 3g; Sodium: 142mg; Cholesterol: 6mg; Total carbs: 36g; Fiber: 2g; Sugar: 33g; Protein: 6g

---

HABIT TRACKER

Did you get 7 to 8 hours of sleep?   ☐ Y ☐ N

Did you drink 2 to 3 liters of water?   ☐ Y   ☐ N
Did you exercise for at least 20 to 30 minutes?   ☐ Y   ☐ N

Today's Big Win: --

Goal(s) for Tomorrow: ---

-

Potassium Punch

Anti-Inflammatory, Brain Health, Heart Health, Immune Boost

SERVES 2

This combo of avocado, banana, and spinach packs a potassium punch, helping your body as it regulates heartbeat and blood pressure. Plus, a diet rich in potassium is important in bone and kidney health, so drink up. The coolest part of this smoothie, though, is that it led me to the discovery of frozen avocado chunks in the market where the other frozen fruit is sold. Nutritious shortcut jackpot!

1 cup unsweetened vanilla almond milk

1 cup baby spinach

1 fresh or frozen banana

½ cup frozen mango

½ cup frozen strawberries

¼ fresh avocado or ¼ cup frozen avocado 1 tablespoon chia seeds

1 tablespoon almond butter

In a blender, combine all the ingredients and blend until the desired consistency is achieved. Add more liquid as needed. Serve immediately.

Ingredient Tip:

Store leftover avocado in the refrigerator, drizzled with a bit of lemon or lime juice to prevent browning or shop online for special avocado storage containers that can help maintain their freshness after cutting.

Per serving:

Calories: 250; Total fat: 12g; Sodium: 93mg; Cholesterol: 0mg; Total

carbs: 33g; Fiber: 9g; Sugar: 17g; Protein: 6g

HABIT TRACKER

Did you get 7 to 8 hours of sleep?   ☐Y ☐N
Did you drink 2 to 3 liters of water?   ☐Y ☐N
Did you exercise for at least 20 to 30 minutes?   ☐Y ☐N
Today's Big Win: ---
Goal(s) for Tomorrow: ---

-

Everything but the . . .

SERVES 2

This smoothie is my take on the kitchen sink, combining a little bit of everything into one filling blend. The high–vitamin C fruits combined with a dose of potassium from spinach and banana make this everything and more when it comes to nutrition in a glass. If you're missing an ingredient or two, just leave it out because this smoothie will still taste delicious.

1 cup skim milk

1 cup baby spinach

1 fresh or frozen banana

¾ cup Siggi's vanilla yogurt

½ cup frozen blueberries ½

cup frozen strawberries ½

cup frozen mango

1 tablespoon hemp seeds

1 tablespoon chia seeds

1 tablespoon rolled oats

In a blender, combine all the ingredients and blend until the desired consistency is achieved. Add more liquid as needed. Serve immediately.

Ingredient Tip:

Siggi's vanilla yogurt is my favorite choice for vanilla yogurt. Not only does it use real sugar but it also uses a lot less than other brands, making it a delicious treat to enjoy anytime.

Per serving:

Calories: 298; Total fat: 9g; Sodium: 122mg; Cholesterol: 14mg; Total carbs: 47g; Fiber: 8g; Sugar: 29g; Protein: 12g

---

HABIT TRACKER

Did you get 7 to 8 hours of sleep?	☐Y ☐N
Did you drink 2 to 3 liters of water?	☐Y ☐N
Did you exercise for at least 20 to 30 minutes?	☐Y ☐N

Today's Big Win: ---

Goal(s) for Tomorrow: --

-

Peach Perfect

Anti-Inflammatory, Digestive Health, Heart Health

SERVES 2

If you haven't seen Pitch Perfect, one of my favorite movies, do yourself a favor and watch it, maybe even while drinking this smoothie. This peachy smoothie is right on pitch with nutrition and taste, and it almost resembles a slice of peach pie with vanilla ice cream melting on top— but without all the added sugar. How good does that sound to satisfy your sweet tooth?

1 cup skim milk

1 cup frozen peaches

1 fresh or frozen banana

¾ cup Siggi's vanilla yogurt

1 tablespoon hemp seeds

Dash ground cinnamon

In a blender, combine all the ingredients and blend until the desired consistency is achieved. Add more liquid as needed. Serve immediately.

Per serving:

Calories: 208; Total fat: 6g; Sodium: 107mg; Cholesterol: 14mg; Total carbs: 32g; Fiber: 3g; Sugar: 24g; Protein: 10g

---

HABIT TRACKER

Did you get 7 to 8 hours of sleep?	☐ Y ☐ N
Did you drink 2 to 3 liters of water?	☐ Y ☐ N

Did you exercise for at least 20 to 30 minutes?   ☐Y ☐N

Today's Big Win: --

Goal(s) for Tomorrow: --

-

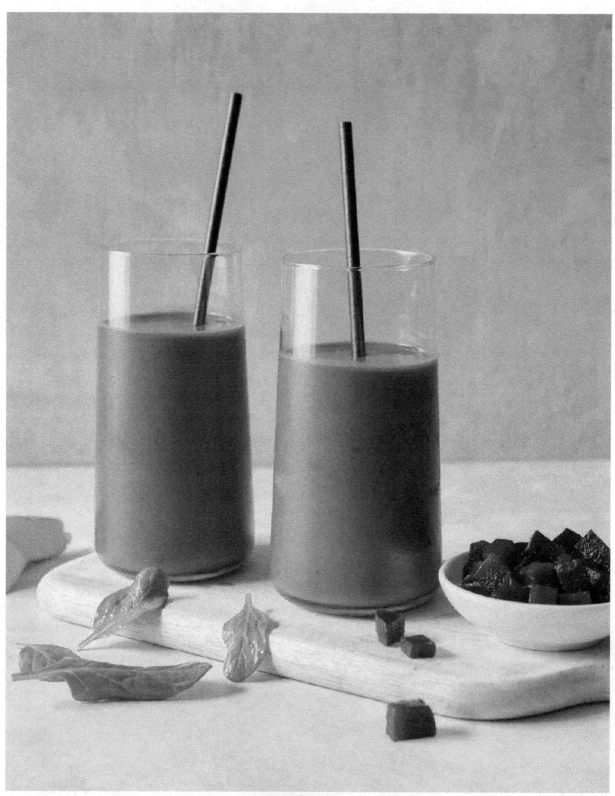

Beet the Bloat

Chapter Five
21-DAY SMOOTHIE SLIM DOWN WEEK 2

HEY, SMOOTHIE LOVERS! I hope your healthy journey to slimming down is going well so far and you're ready for more smoothie-tastic goodness. Remember to keep your head up and be positive and patient so that your habits begin to naturally adjust and you realize just how good your mind and body are supposed to feel when you focus on a diet filled with quality, nutrient-dense foods. I created these recipes so that you have a handful of quick, flexible meal options each week using more or less the same ingredients as the previous week. The perks of using frozen fruit are that it doesn't spoil like fresh fruit, you can always have it on hand in your freezer, and it can be a more economical option. The fewer trips to the grocery store, the better! So, break out that blender and let's continue to work on the shinier, healthier version of you that is dying to come out and say hello—with a smoothie in hand, of course.

WEEK 2 SHOPPING LIST

FRUITS AND VEGETABLES

- Avocado (1)
- Bananas (4)
- Kale (1 cup)
- Lime (1)
- Oranges, mandarin (2)
- Spinach, baby (3 cups)

FROZEN

- Berries, mixed (1 cup)
- Blueberries (½ cup)
- Cauliflower, riced (½ cup)
- Cherries (1 cup)
- Peaches (1 cup)
- Pineapple (2 cups)
- Strawberries (2½ cups)
- Tropical fruit mix (1 cup)

MILKS, NONDAIRY MILKS, AND YOGURTS

- Almond milk, unsweetened vanilla (1 [32-ounce] container)
- Coconut milk, unsweetened (refrigerated, not canned) (16 ounces)
- Dairy milk, skim or low-fat (1 [8-ounce] container)
- Yogurt, nonfat or low-fat plain Greek or Icelandic (1 [16-ounce]

container)

- Yogurt, Siggi's low-fat or whole-milk vanilla (1 [24-ounce] container)
- Yogurt, unsweetened plain coconut (1 [16-ounce] container)

PANTRY

- Almond butter
- Cacao powder
- Chia seeds
- Cinnamon, ground
- Coffee
- Hemp seeds
- Mini dark chocolate chips (optional)

Piña Mama

Anti-Inflammatory, Digestive Health, Heart Health, Immune Boost

SERVES 2

If you like piña coladas and getting caught in the rain, then this is a healthy treat that is right in your lane. A boost of filling, fiber-rich chia seeds rounds out this tropical mix.

1 cup unsweetened coconut milk

1 cup frozen pineapple

1 cup frozen strawberries

¾ cup plain coconut yogurt

1 tablespoon chia seeds

In a blender, combine all the ingredients and blend until the desired consistency is achieved. Add more liquid as needed. Serve immediately.

Bonus Boost:

Pineapples contain tons of nutrients and antioxidants, plus a group of enzymes known as bromelain that not only ease digestion but also have properties that may help alleviate symptoms of inflammatory diseases such as arthritis.

Per serving:

Calories: 200; Total fat: 6g; Sodium: 122mg; Cholesterol: 0mg; Total carbs: 29g; Fiber: 6g; Sugar: 18g; Protein: 6g

HABIT TRACKER
Did you get 7 to 8 hours of sleep?   ☐ Y ☐ N

Did you drink 2 to 3 liters of water?   ☐ Y   ☐ N

Did you exercise for at least 20 to 30 minutes?   ☐ Y   ☐ N

Today's Big Win: --

Goal(s) for Tomorrow: ---

-

An AB&J a Day Keeps the Doctor Away

Heart Health

SERVES 2

You complete me, nut butter. If I could only take one item to a deserted island with me, it would be nut butter. I literally eat a version of this treat every day. Okay, you get the point. The classic PB&J gets an upgrade with heart-healthy almond butter blended with fiber-rich berries and spinach. I often add a banana to my sandwiches for an extra boost of sweetness and substance.

1 cup unsweetened vanilla almond milk

1 cup frozen mixed berries

1 cup baby spinach

1 fresh or frozen banana

2 tablespoons almond butter

In a blender, combine all the ingredients and blend until the desired consistency is achieved. Add more liquid as needed. Serve immediately.

Per serving:

Calories: 209; Total fat: 11g; Sodium: 90mg; Cholesterol: 0mg; Total carbs: 27g; Fiber: 6g; Sugar: 16g; Protein: 5g

HABIT TRACKER

Did you get 7 to 8 hours of sleep?   ☐ Y ☐ N

Did you drink 2 to 3 liters of water?   ☐ Y ☐ N

Did you exercise for at least 20 to 30 minutes? ☐Y ☐N

Today's Big Win: --

Goal(s) for Tomorrow: --

-

Breakfast Margarita

Anti-Inflammatory, Heart Health, Immune Boost

SERVES 2

Margaritas can have a place at the breakfast table, too, as long as you mocktail it and hold the tequila. Just pretend, because it will be 5 o'clock sooner or later. This strawberry margarita combines vitamin C– rich berries, oranges, and lime juice for a refreshing blend of nutritious fruity ingredients.

1 cup unsweetened coconut milk

1 cup frozen strawberries

2 mandarin oranges

¾ cup plain coconut yogurt

¼ fresh avocado or ¼ cup frozen

avocado Juice of ½ lime

1 tablespoon hemp seeds

In a blender, combine all the ingredients and blend until the desired consistency is achieved. Add more liquid as needed. Serve immediately.

Bonus Boost:

Avocado, coconut yogurt, and coconut milk provide heart-healthy fats and add a hit of electrolytes for a hydrating start to your day.

Per serving:

Calories: 254; Total fat: 8g; Sodium: 143mg; Cholesterol: 0mg; Total

carbs: 38g; Fiber: 8g; Sugar: 26g; Protein: 8g

HABIT TRACKER

Did you get 7 to 8 hours of sleep?   ☐Y ☐N
Did you drink 2 to 3 liters of water?   ☐Y ☐N
Did you exercise for at least 20 to 30 minutes?   ☐Y ☐N

Today's Big Win: ---

Goal(s) for Tomorrow: --

-

LBN Slims Vanilla Latte

Anti-Inflammatory, Heart Health

SERVES 2

I don't know about you but the ritual of sitting in a neighborhood coffee shop and enjoying a vanilla latte makes me happy. It's the little things in life. This frozen version still creates that cozy feeling but it's satiating enough for a meal or snack due to its protein and fiber-rich blend of fruit, seeds, and yogurt. Save leftover coffee in a jar and store in the refrigerator for smoothie additions or for an anytime iced coffee!

2 fresh or frozen bananas

¾ cup Siggi's vanilla

yogurt 4 ice cubes

½ cup leftover coffee

½ cup unsweetened vanilla almond

milk 1 tablespoon chia seeds

Dash ground cinnamon

In a blender, combine all the ingredients and blend until the desired consistency is achieved. Add more liquid as needed. Serve immediately.

Per serving:

Calories: 211; Total fat: 4g; Sodium: 102mg; Cholesterol: 5mg; Total carbs: 40g; Fiber: 6g; Sugar: 25g; Protein: 7g

HABIT TRACKER

Did you get 7 to 8 hours of sleep?	☐ Y ☐ N
Did you drink 2 to 3 liters of water?	☐ Y ☐ N

Did you exercise for at least 20 to 30 minutes? ☐Y ☐N

Today's Big Win: --

Goal(s) for Tomorrow: --

-

Life Is but a Green

Anti-Inflammatory, Brain Health, Digestive Health, Immune Boost

SERVES 2

This smoothie might appear greenish but don't be squeamish. You would never know there are superfood greens blended up with sweet tropical fruits in this dreamy treat. Greek yogurt and hemp seeds add nutritious protein and fat that keep your mind and belly relaxed and satisfied. If you don't have kale, substitute another cup of baby spinach instead.

1 cup unsweetened vanilla almond milk

1 cup frozen tropical fruit mix

1 cup frozen pineapple

1 cup baby spinach

1 cup kale

¾ cup plain low-fat Greek yogurt

1 tablespoon hemp seeds

In a blender, combine all the ingredients and blend until the desired consistency is achieved. Add more liquid as needed. Serve immediately.

Per serving:

Calories: 263; Total fat: 5g; Sodium: 159mg; Cholesterol: 6mg; Total carbs: 49g; Fiber: 4g; Sugar: 16g; Protein: 8g

HABIT TRACKER

Did you get 7 to 8 hours of sleep?	☐ Y ☐ N
Did you drink 2 to 3 liters of water?	☐ Y ☐ N

Did you exercise for at least 20 to 30 minutes?   ☐Y ☐N

Today's Big Win: --

Goal(s) for Tomorrow: --

-

Dark Chocolate Star

Anti-Inflammatory, Heart Health, Immune Boost

SERVES 2

Soar through the sky—I mean your busy day—with a double dose of chocolatey milkshake goodness that will lighten up your mood and 'tude. Chocolate chips on top are optional but always highly recommended in my galaxy.

1 cup skim milk

1 cup frozen cherries

1 cup frozen peaches

1 cup baby spinach

¾ cup Siggi's vanilla yogurt

1 tablespoon chia seeds

1 tablespoon cacao powder

Mini dark chocolate chips, for serving (optional)

In a blender, combine all the ingredients (except the optional chocolate chips) and blend until the desired consistency is achieved. Add more liquid as needed. Sprinkle the chocolate chips (if using) on top and serve immediately.

Bonus Boost:

Fruits and spinach kick up the vitamin C and antioxidants and the yogurt and milk add protein and a creamy texture.

Per serving:

Calories: 210; Total fat: 3g; Sodium: 141mg; Cholesterol: 4mg; Total

carbs: 35g; Fiber: 6g; Sugar: 27g; Protein: 13g

HABIT TRACKER

Did you get 7 to 8 hours of sleep?   ☐Y ☐N

Did you drink 2 to 3 liters of water?   ☐Y ☐N

Did you exercise for at least 20 to 30 minutes?   ☐Y ☐N

Today's Big Win: --

Goal(s) for Tomorrow: ---

-

Colonel Cauli

Anti-Inflammatory, Heart Health, Immune Boost

SERVES 2

I do like cauliflower in my smoothies—sir, yes, sir! What a surprise, I have discovered another use for the almighty cauliflower in your diet. The truth of the matter is, the addition of this powerhouse cruciferous veggie not only adds a boost of vitamins, minerals, fiber, and antioxidants to a blend of already nutritious fruits, but it also brings a delightful frosty texture to any smoothie. Talk about hidden talent. This veggie does it all!

1 cup unsweetened vanilla almond milk

1 fresh or frozen banana

¾ cup plain low-fat Greek

yogurt ½ cup frozen blueberries

½ cup frozen strawberries

½ cup frozen riced cauliflower

1 tablespoon hemp seeds

In a blender, combine all the ingredients and blend until the desired consistency is achieved. Add more liquid as needed. Serve immediately.

Per serving:

Calories: 204; Total fat: 5g; Sodium: 142mg; Cholesterol: 6mg; Total carbs: 33g; Fiber: 5g; Sugar: 22g; Protein: 8g

HABIT TRACKER
Did you get 7 to 8 hours of sleep?   ☐ Y ☐ N

Did you drink 2 to 3 liters of water?   ☐ Y   ☐ N
Did you exercise for at least 20 to 30 minutes?   ☐ Y   ☐ N

Today's Big Win: --

Goal(s) for Tomorrow: --

-

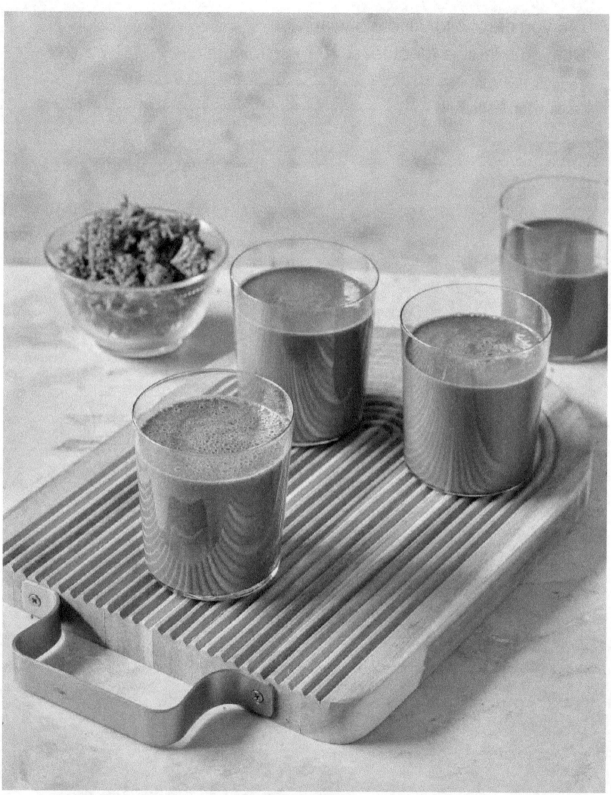

Gene's Green Machine

Chapter Six
21-DAY SMOOTHIE SLIM DOWN WEEK 3

BY NOW YOU SHOULD BE FEELING lighter and more confident in your choices, so give yourself a big hug and let's move forward. Think of the positive changes you have made in the first few weeks and remember to keep in mind that change takes time and persistence. It's all too easy to let life get in the way of staying consistent with healthy choices but imagine how great you will look and feel if you commit to a lifestyle that will ultimately add years to your life. Your body will reward you when you put in the work, but please anticipate the fact that not all days will look like the colorful pictures of pretty smoothies in this book. Real life presents plenty of struggles, but when you push through them, your mind-set and choices improve and help you on your path to a healthier life. Start your smoothie engines because it's week 3!

WEEK 3 SHOPPING LIST

FRUITS AND VEGETABLES

- Avocado (1)
- Bananas (2)
- Kale (2 cups)
- Spinach, baby (2 cups)

FROZEN

- Berries, mixed (1 cup)
- Blackberries (1 cup)
- Blueberries (1 cup)
- Cauliflower, riced (½ cup)
- Cherries (2 cups)
- Dragon fruit (1 [3.5-ounce] packet)
- Mangos (3½ cups)
- Peaches (½ cup)
- Pineapple (½ cup)
- Strawberries (½ cup)
- Tropical fruit mix (1 cup)

MILKS, NONDAIRY MILKS, AND YOGURTS

- Almond milk, unsweetened vanilla (1 [32-ounce] container)
- Coconut milk, unsweetened (refrigerated, not canned) (16 ounces)
- Dairy milk, skim or low-fat (1 [8-ounce] container)

- Yogurt, nonfat or low-fat plain Greek or Icelandic (1 [32-ounce] container)
- Yogurt, Siggi's low-fat or whole-milk vanilla (2 [4.4-ounce] containers)
- Yogurt, unsweetened plain coconut (1 [16-ounce] container)

PANTRY

- Cacao powder
- Chia seeds
- Cinnamon, ground
- Coffee
- Hemp seeds

Berry Good Batch

Anti-Inflammatory, Heart Health, Immune Boost

SERVES 2

You'll feel berry good after blending up this batch of fiber-rich berries and sweet mango with nutritious but undetectable kale. Greek yogurt and chia seeds boost the protein and healthy fat profile.

1 cup unsweetened vanilla almond milk

1 cup frozen mixed berries

1 cup frozen mango

1 cup kale

¾ cup plain low-fat Greek

yogurt 1 tablespoon chia seeds

In a blender, combine all the ingredients and blend until the desired consistency is achieved. Add more liquid as needed. Serve immediately.

Per serving:

Calories: 197; Total fat: 5g; Sodium: 146mg; Cholesterol: 6mg; Total carbs: 30g; Fiber: 6g; Sugar: 23g; Protein: 8g

---

HABIT TRACKER

Did you get 7 to 8 hours of sleep?	☐ Y ☐ N
Did you drink 2 to 3 liters of water?	☐ Y ☐ N
Did you exercise for at least 20 to 30 minutes?	☐ Y ☐ N

Today's Big Win: --

Goal(s) for Tomorrow: --

Gene's Green Machine

Anti-Inflammatory, Brain Health, Heart Health

SERVES 2

This green blend will turn you into an energized machine that can take on the world, or perhaps just fix something in your house today. The sweet mango and banana mask the taste of green powerhouse gems spinach and avocado for a refreshing mix of vitamins, minerals, and healthy fats.

1 cup unsweetened coconut milk

1 cup frozen mango

1 cup baby spinach

1 fresh or frozen banana

¾ cup plain coconut yogurt

¼ fresh avocado or ¼ cup frozen avocado

In a blender, combine all the ingredients and blend until the desired consistency is achieved. Add more liquid as needed. Serve immediately.

Bonus Boost:

Avocados are one of the best sources of monounsaturated heart-healthy fats and one of my favorite (and tastiest!) ways to add a boatload of nutrition into any diet. If I don't eat some at least once a day, I don't feel complete.

Per serving:

Calories: 222; Total fat: 9g; Sodium: 133mg; Cholesterol: 0mg; Total carbs: 34g; Fiber: 5g; Sugar: 25g; Protein: 6g

HABIT TRACKER

Did you get 7 to 8 hours of sleep?   ☐Y ☐N

Did you drink 2 to 3 liters of water?   ☐Y ☐N

Did you exercise for at least 20 to 30 minutes?   ☐Y ☐N

Today's Big Win: ---

Goal(s) for Tomorrow: ---

-

Pink Paradise

Anti-Inflammatory, Heart Health

SERVES 2

Dragon fruit stars again in this fruity smoothie and provides the bright pink color and antioxidants that will put a little pep in your pink-smoothie step. Protein-packed Greek yogurt and chia seeds make this smoothie a pinkalicious meal.

1 cup unsweetened vanilla almond milk

1 cup frozen mango

¾ cup plain low-fat Greek yogurt

1 (3.5-ounce) packet frozen dragon fruit

1 tablespoon chia seeds

In a blender, combine all the ingredients and blend until the desired consistency is achieved. Add more liquid as needed. Serve immediately.

Per serving:

Calories: 196; Total fat: 5g; Sodium: 142mg; Cholesterol: 6mg; Total carbs: 31g; Fiber: 6g; Sugar: 24g; Protein: 7g

---

HABIT TRACKER

Did you get 7 to 8 hours of sleep?	☐ Y	☐ N
Did you drink 2 to 3 liters of water?	☐ Y	☐ N
Did you exercise for at least 20 to 30 minutes?	☐ Y	☐ N

Today's Big Win: --

Goal(s) for Tomorrow: --

-

Summer Shake-Up

Anti-Inflammatory, Digestive Health, Heart Health

SERVES 2

Shake it up in any season with this mix of summer fruits that are available in the freezer all year long. Vanilla yogurt combines with the nuttiness of hemp seeds and the sweet spice of cinnamon to create a fantastic flavor that tastes like a fruit cobbler with a scoop of creamy vanilla on top.

1 cup frozen blackberries

¾ cup Siggi's whole-milk vanilla yogurt

½ cup unsweetened vanilla almond

milk ½ cup frozen strawberries

½ cup frozen peaches

1 tablespoon hemp seeds

Dash ground cinnamon

In a blender, combine all the ingredients and blend until the desired consistency is achieved. Add more liquid as needed. Serve immediately.

Per serving:

Calories: 187; Total fat: 6g; Sodium: 82mg; Cholesterol: 12mg; Total carbs: 23g; Fiber: 6g; Sugar: 16g; Protein: 6g

HABIT TRACKER

Did you get 7 to 8 hours of sleep?	☐ Y ☐ N
Did you drink 2 to 3 liters of water?	☐ Y ☐ N
Did you exercise for at least 20 to 30 minutes?	☐ Y ☐ N

Today's Big Win: --

Goal(s) for Tomorrow: --

-

Mercer Built Mocha

Heart Health

SERVES 2

If the awesome team at Mercer Built can build your dream house, then I can build your dream smoothie with a mocha twist. When you combine antioxidant-rich sweet cherries and banana with a hint of chocolate and coffee, you will feel like you're enjoying a luxurious treat, but this blend contains zero added sugar thanks to real cacao powder and black coffee.

1 fresh or frozen banana

1 cup frozen cherries

1 cup baby spinach

¾ cup plain low-fat Greek

yogurt ½ cup skim milk

½ cup leftover coffee

1 tablespoon cacao powder

In a blender, combine all the ingredients and blend until the desired consistency is achieved. Add more liquid as needed. Serve immediately.

Per serving:

Calories: 178; Total fat: 3g; Sodium: 111mg; Cholesterol: 7mg; Total carbs: 34g; Fiber: 4g; Sugar: 24g; Protein: 9g

HABIT TRACKER

Did you get 7 to 8 hours of sleep?	☐ Y ☐ N
Did you drink 2 to 3 liters of water?	☐ Y ☐ N

Did you exercise for at least 20 to 30 minutes?   ☐Y ☐N

Today's Big Win: ---

Goal(s) for Tomorrow: ---

-

Clueless Cauli

Anti-Inflammatory, Brain Health, Digestive Health, Heart Health, Immune Boost

SERVES 2

You'll be clueless that this tasty fruit trio does the tango with frozen cauliflower. Just remember that you are welcome to add cauliflower to any smoothie to bump up the nutrition without ever knowing this cruciferous friend is blended up in the mix. As Cher from Clueless (my favorite movie) would say, "As if!"

1 cup unsweetened coconut milk

1 cup frozen blueberries

¾ cup plain coconut yogurt

½ cup frozen pineapple ½

cup frozen mango

½ cup frozen riced cauliflower

1 tablespoon chia seeds

In a blender, combine all the ingredients and blend until the desired consistency is achieved. Add more liquid as needed. Serve immediately.

Bonus Boost:

Cauliflower is everywhere for a reason and it's not going anywhere! Not only is it versatile and full of fiber and nutrients, but it is also one of the best low-calorie and low-carb alternatives to grains and pasta and adds texture and volume to any smoothie or meal so you stay full and satisfied.

Per serving:

Calories: 209; Total fat: 7g; Sodium: 129mg; Cholesterol: 0mg; Total

carbs: 31g; Fiber: 7g; Sugar: 23g; Protein: 6g

HABIT TRACKER

Did you get 7 to 8 hours of sleep?   ☐Y ☐N

Did you drink 2 to 3 liters of water?   ☐Y ☐N

Did you exercise for at least 20 to 30 minutes?   ☐Y ☐N

Today's Big Win: ---

Goal(s) for Tomorrow: --

-

Chocoholic

Anti-Inflammatory, Brain Health, Digestive Health, Heart Health, Immune Boost

SERVES 2

There's no shame in my love for chocolate game. A hit of chocolatey yet antioxidant-rich cacao powder blended with the natural sweetness from tropical fruit and cherries creates this chocolicious smoothie.

1 cup unsweetened vanilla almond milk

1 cup frozen tropical fruit mix

1 cup frozen cherries

1 cup kale

¾ cup plain low-fat Greek yogurt

1 tablespoon cacao powder

1 tablespoon hemp seeds

In a blender, combine all the ingredients and blend until the desired consistency is achieved. Add more liquid as needed. Serve immediately.

Per serving:

Calories: 209; Total fat: 8g; Sodium: 123mg; Cholesterol: 12mg; Total carbs: 30g; Fiber: 6g; Sugar: 23g; Protein: 7g

HABIT TRACKER

Did you get 7 to 8 hours of sleep?	☐ Y	☐ N
Did you drink 2 to 3 liters of water?	☐ Y	☐ N
Did you exercise for at least 20 to 30 minutes?	☐ Y	☐ N

Today's Big Win: --

Goal(s) for Tomorrow: ---
-

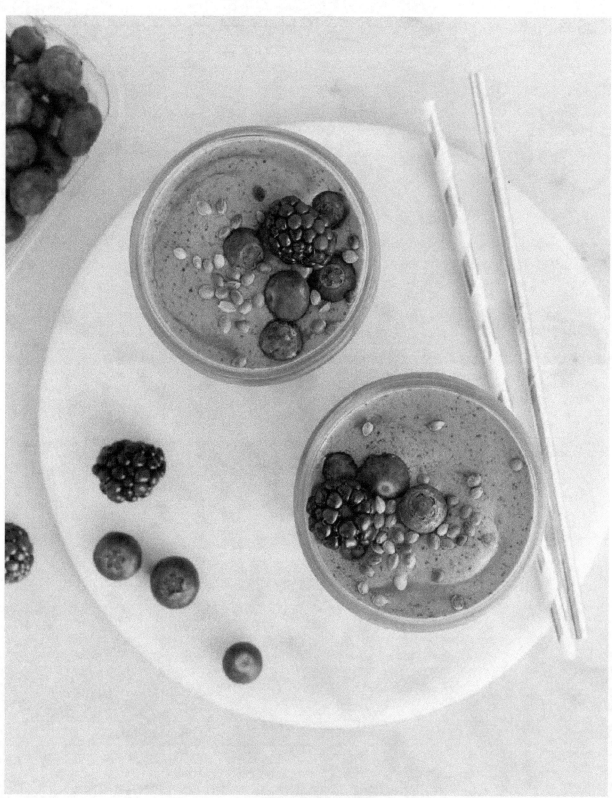

LB's Blissed-Out Berries

Chapter Seven
7-DAY DETOX

DO YOU WANT TO HEAR SOMETHING COOL? Even though this week is labeled as a "detox," your body has its own super-powerful system for naturally detoxing your body all the time! The main organs involved are your liver and kidneys, and they work very well to "cleanse" your body, so please don't subscribe to any uber-restrictive diet plans that claim to magically detox you. Most of these plans or liquid-only programs are simply starvation diets that are not only silly and short-lived but unhealthy for your mind and body's metabolic needs. Instead, let's rephrase this plan to something responsible and more legit, like a debloat week, so that you can feel better quickly after a rough patch. If you've ever slipped from your healthy habits for a while (nah, that never happens), and you have that puffy or heavy feeling from too much of everything, then this week of smoothies is your food prescription. These blends contain special ingredients that help your body naturally detox and let go of excess water and sodium, which tend to be the main culprits in that icky feeling. Remember, in order to reap the full benefits and feel your best, it is even more important that you couple this week (and beyond) with healthier lifestyle habits like drinking enough water, refraining from excess alcohol intake, stressing less, sleeping more, and limiting the processed packaged foods in your diet that contain added sugar and sodium. During this week, feel free to sub in an extra smoothie for a meal, add as many veggies as you can, and focus on a light dinner. Use this bonus week not only to beat the bloat and mentally reset but to jump-start your healthier future.

7-DAY DETOX SHOPPING LIST

FRUITS AND VEGETABLES

- Bananas (3)
- Beet (1)
- Ginger root (1 [2-inch] piece) (optional)
- Kale (1 cup)
- Kiwis (5)
- Lemons (2)
- Spinach, baby (5 cups)

FROZEN

- Berries, mixed (2 cups)
- Cauliflower, riced (½ cup)
- Mangos (2½ cups)
- Pineapple (3 cups)
- Strawberries (1½ cups)

MILKS, NONDAIRY MILKS, AND YOGURTS

- Almond milk, unsweetened vanilla (1 [32-ounce] container)
- Coconut milk, unsweetened (refrigerated, not canned) (20 ounces)
- Yogurt, nonfat or low-fat plain Greek or Icelandic (1 [32-ounce] container)
- Yogurt, unsweetened plain coconut (1 [24-ounce] container)

PANTRY

- Black pepper, freshly ground
- Chia seeds
- Cinnamon, ground
- Ginger, ground
- Turmeric, ground

Georgie's Ginger Gem

Anti-Inflammatory, Brain Health, Digestive Health, Heart Health, Immune Boost

SERVES 2

George, turn up the smoothie bass! Named after our bassist friend George, this smoothie is packed with potassium, antioxidants, and a nice hit of spicy, anti-inflammatory ginger. This blend of fruits and greens is the perfect gem for kicking off a jump-start week of naturally debloating your system so it sings beautifully again.

1 cup unsweetened coconut milk

1 cup frozen mango

1 cup kale

1 fresh or frozen banana

¾ cup plain coconut

yogurt Juice of 1 lemon

1 tablespoon chia seeds

1 tablespoon fresh ginger or 2 teaspoons ground ginger

In a blender, combine all the ingredients and blend until the desired consistency is achieved. Add more liquid as needed. Serve immediately.

Bonus Boost:

Ginger is warming and can stimulate digestion, boost circulation, and even help ease arthritic pain, so be sure not to skip this small but mighty addition in your smoothie.

Per serving:

Calories: 225; Total fat: 7g; Sodium: 124mg; Cholesterol: 0mg; Total

carbs: 37g; Fiber: 6g; Sugar: 25g; Protein: 7g

HABIT TRACKER

Did you get 7 to 8 hours of sleep?   ☐Y ☐N

Did you drink 2 to 3 liters of water?   ☐Y ☐N

Did you exercise for at least 20 to 30 minutes?   ☐Y ☐N

Today's Big Win: --

Goal(s) for Tomorrow: ---

-

Tie-Dye Turmeric Twist

Anti-Inflammatory, Brain Health, Digestive Health, Heart Health, Immune Boost

SERVES 2

Tie-dye is all the rage, so let's twist it up with a colorful concoction of bright fruits, veggies, and spices. No artificial anything is needed when Mother Nature's ingredients provide bursts of color. Curcumin is the strong anti-inflammatory compound in turmeric and black pepper and when they're combined, they're absorbed much better. So don't think I'm crazy for adding pepper to a smoothie!

1 cup unsweetened coconut milk

1 cup frozen mixed berries

1 cup frozen pineapple

1 cup baby spinach or kale

¾ cup plain coconut yogurt

1 teaspoon ground turmeric

1 teaspoon ground cinnamon

Dash freshly ground black pepper

In a blender, combine all the ingredients and blend until the desired consistency is achieved. Add more liquid as needed. Serve immediately.

Per serving:

Calories: 171; Total fat: 5g; Sodium: 124mg; Cholesterol: 0mg; Total carbs: 29g; Fiber: 5g; Sugar: 19g; Protein: 5g

HABIT TRACKER
Did you get 7 to 8 hours of sleep?   ☐ Y ☐ N

Did you drink 2 to 3 liters of water? ☐ Y ☐ N

Did you exercise for at least 20 to 30 minutes? ☐ Y ☐ N

Today's Big Win: ---

Goal(s) for Tomorrow: ---

-

Krazy Kiwi

Anti-Inflammatory, Brain Health, Digestive Health, Heart Health, Immune Boost

SERVES 2

Who knew a hairy green fruit could be so nutritious, delicious, and naturally detoxifying? Don't judge a book by its cover because kiwis win the prize for the fruit with the most amount of vitamin C and fiber in the littlest package.

1 cup unsweetened vanilla almond milk

1 cup baby spinach or kale

2 whole kiwis

¾ cup plain low-fat Greek yogurt

½ cup frozen strawberries

½ cup frozen mango

1 tablespoon chia seeds

In a blender, combine all the ingredients and blend until the desired consistency is achieved. Add more liquid as needed. Serve immediately.

Ingredient Tip:

The skin of kiwi fruit is edible, so toss the whole kiwi in, peel and all, for the easiest smoothie prep around.

Per serving:

Calories: 203; Total fat: 5g; Sodium: 148mg; Cholesterol: 6mg; Total carbs: 32g; Fiber: 7g; Sugar: 22g; Protein: 8g

HABIT TRACKER

Did you get 7 to 8 hours of sleep?   ☐ Y   ☐ N

Did you drink 2 to 3 liters of water?   ☐ Y   ☐ N

Did you exercise for at least 20 to 30 minutes?   ☐ Y   ☐ N

Today's Big Win: ---

Goal(s) for Tomorrow: --

-

Bart's Green Banana

Anti-Inflammatory, Brain Health, Digestive Health, Heart Health, Immune Boost

SERVES 2

The Bart family lives life to the absolute fullest and can turn even green food into a culinary masterpiece. Beat the bloat with this sweet but green blend of fruits and veggies that provides a hefty dose of potassium and hydrating coconut. Cinnamon and cha-cha-chia bump up the nutrition factor with heart-healthy properties.

1 cup baby spinach or kale

1 fresh or frozen banana

2 whole kiwis

¾ cup plain coconut

yogurt 4 ice cubes

½ cup unsweetened coconut

milk 1 tablespoon chia seeds

Dash ground cinnamon

In a blender, combine all the ingredients and blend until the desired consistency is achieved. Add more liquid as needed. Serve immediately.

Per serving:

Calories: 187; Total fat: 6g; Sodium: 87mg; Cholesterol: 0mg; Total carbs: 28g; Fiber: 7g; Sugar: 15g; Protein: 7g

---

HABIT TRACKER

Did you get 7 to 8 hours of sleep?   ☐ Y ☐ N

Did you drink 2 to 3 liters of water?   ☐ Y ☐ N

Did you exercise for at least 20 to 30 minutes?   ☐Y ☐N

Today's Big Win: ---

Goal(s) for Tomorrow: --

-

Yellow Yogi

Anti-Inflammatory, Digestive Health, Heart Health, Immune Boost

SERVES 2

Get ready to "namastay" happy all week when you calm your mind and body with this hydrating blend of bright yellow fruits and antioxidant-rich turmeric. This combo of ingredients is a zen recipe for creating peace and harmony in your body.

1 cup unsweetened vanilla almond milk

1 cup frozen mango

1 cup frozen pineapple

¾ cup plain low-fat Greek

yogurt Juice of ½ lemon

1 tablespoon chia seeds

1 teaspoon ground turmeric

Dash freshly ground black pepper

In a blender, combine all the ingredients and blend until the desired consistency is achieved. Add more liquid as needed. Serve immediately.

Bonus Boost:

The dash of black pepper will increase the absorption of turmeric, so give it a go!

Per serving:

Calories: 210; Total fat: 5g; Sodium: 143mg; Cholesterol: 6mg; Total

carbs: 35g; Fiber: 6g; Sugar: 28g; Protein: 8g

HABIT TRACKER

Did you get 7 to 8 hours of sleep?   ☐Y ☐N

Did you drink 2 to 3 liters of water?   ☐Y ☐N

Did you exercise for at least 20 to 30 minutes?   ☐Y ☐N

Today's Big Win: ---

Goal(s) for Tomorrow: ---

-

Beet the Bloat

Anti-Inflammatory, Brain Health, Digestive Health, Heart Health, Immune Boost

SERVES 2

Banish that bloated feeling with the superfood duo of beets and ginger. This ripe-red blend combines fiber-rich beets and berries with sweet pineapple to balance out the flavors. If you're wondering what to do if you don't own a high-speed blender, let me beet you to the answer: Boil or microwave the raw beets first.

1 cup unsweetened vanilla almond milk

1 small beet, cubed, or 1 cup frozen beets

1 cup frozen mixed berries

1 cup frozen pineapple

1 cup baby spinach or kale

¾ cup plain low-fat Greek

yogurt 1 tablespoon chia seeds

1 tablespoon fresh ginger or 2 teaspoons ground ginger

In a blender, combine all the ingredients and blend until the desired consistency is achieved. Add more liquid as needed. Serve immediately.

Per serving:

Calories: 201; Total fat: 5g; Sodium: 178mg; Cholesterol: 6mg; Total carbs: 32g; Fiber: 7g; Sugar: 23g; Protein: 8g

---

HABIT TRACKER

Did you get 7 to 8 hours of sleep?   ☐ Y ☐ N

Did you drink 2 to 3 liters of water?   ☐ Y ☐ N

Did you exercise for at least 20 to 30 minutes?　　　☐Y ☐N

Today's Big Win: ---

Goal(s) for Tomorrow: ---

-

Caul Me Strawberry Slims

Anti-Inflammatory, Heart Health, Immune Boost

SERVES 2

Hello again, my nutritious cauliflower friend. The extra boost of fiber, nutrition, and frostiness from this hidden veggie blended with a trio of potassium-rich fruits is a recipe for feeling slimmer even sooner.

1 cup unsweetened vanilla almond milk

1 cup frozen strawberries

1 cup baby spinach or kale

1 fresh or frozen banana

¾ cup plain low-fat Greek

yogurt 1 whole kiwi

½ cup frozen riced cauliflower

1 tablespoon chia seeds

In a blender, combine all the ingredients and blend until the desired consistency is achieved. Add more liquid as needed. Serve immediately.

Per serving:

Calories: 236; Total fat: 5g; Sodium: 121mg; Cholesterol: 6mg; Total carbs: 39g; Fiber: 8g; Sugar: 23g; Protein: 9g

---

HABIT TRACKER

Did you get 7 to 8 hours of sleep?	☐ Y	☐ N
Did you drink 2 to 3 liters of water?	☐ Y	☐ N
Did you exercise for at least 20 to 30 minutes?	☐ Y	☐ N

Today's Big Win: --
Goal(s) for Tomorrow: --

-

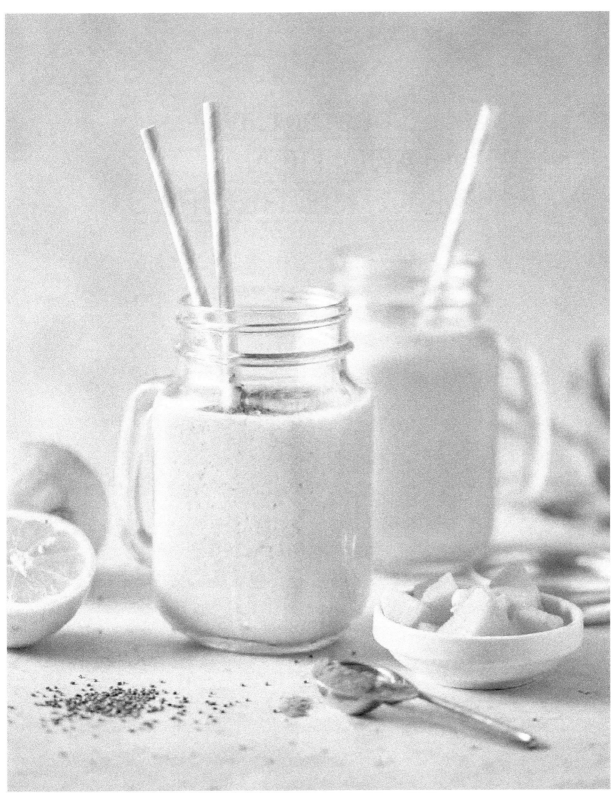

Orange You Glad (This Is the Last Smoothie)!

Chapter Eight
ADDITIONAL
SMOOTHIE RECIPES

Margate Morning Dew

Heart Health, Immune Boost

SERVES 2

There's nothing like the sight of morning dew and the smell of saltwater in the summer when I am in my happy place at the Jersey Shore in Margate with this smoothie in hand. Honeydew is not only sweet and refreshing but also has a strong nutrient profile as a solid source of vitamin C, which is essential for immune support and skin repair. Raspberries and spinach add even more vitamin C, antioxidants, and fiber to this energizing eye-opener.

1 cup unsweetened vanilla almond milk

1 cup honeydew melon

1 cup frozen raspberries

1 cup plain low-fat Greek yogurt

1 cup baby spinach

1 tablespoon chia seeds

In a blender, combine all the ingredients and blend until the desired consistency is achieved. Add more liquid as needed. Serve immediately.

Bonus Boost:

Honeydew contains the bone-building nutrients folate, vitamin K, and magnesium.

Per serving:

Calories: 208; Total fat: 6g; Sodium: 191mg; Cholesterol: 7mg; Total carbs: 29g; Fiber: 9g; Sugar: 20g; Protein: 10g

The Wise Watermelon

Anti-Inflammatory, Brain Health, Heart Health, Immune Boost

SERVES 2

Watermelon is a great source of lycopene, which is a strong antioxidant that prevents cell damage. Because lycopene is fat soluble, it is absorbed better when blended with fat sources like the coconut and chia seeds in this smoothie.

1½ cups chopped watermelon

1 cup unsweetened coconut milk

1 cup frozen strawberries

1 cup frozen riced cauliflower

1 cup plain coconut yogurt

1 tablespoon chia seeds

In a blender, combine all the ingredients and blend until the desired consistency is achieved. Add more liquid as needed. Serve immediately.

Bonus Boost:

Riced cauliflower boosts the vitamin C and fiber content even more, and you won't even know it's hiding in there! Fat from coconut is great for your melon, so wise up and try this one.

Per serving:

Calories: 229; Total fat: 8g; Sodium: 142mg; Cholesterol: 0mg; Total carbs: 32g; Fiber: 7g; Sugar: 20g; Protein: 8g

Cherries Joybilee

Anti-Inflammatory, Heart Health, Immune Boost

SERVES 2

This simple combo of sweet cherries and protein-packed plain yogurt with a hint of vanilla is the perfect shake for a pre- or post-workout snack or a light snack before bedtime. My former boss and mentor Joy Bauer is excellent at explaining nutrition in the most relatable way and bringing joy to the Today Show audience on a daily basis, so she would make sure to tell you that cherries contain anti-inflammatory and antioxidant properties that may help with such ailments as arthritis and gout. Oh Joy!

2 cups frozen dark cherries

1 cup skim milk

1 cup plain low-fat Greek yogurt

1 teaspoon vanilla extract

In a blender, combine all the ingredients and blend until the desired consistency is achieved. Add more liquid as needed. Serve immediately.

Bonus Boost:

Cherries are loaded with vitamin C and rich in anthocyanins, a strong anti-inflammatory, antioxidant, and pain-relieving compound.

Per serving:

Calories: 198; Total fat: 3g; Sodium: 152mg; Cholesterol: 10mg; Total carbs: 32g; Fiber: 3g; Sugar: 29g; Protein: 12g

The Green Berry Banana

Anti-Inflammatory, Heart Health, Immune Boost

SERVES 2

The fruits and spinach in this green smoothie combine the powers of potassium and vitamin C for an immunity-boosting blend. The Greek yogurt packs a high-protein punch and creates a super creamy consistency.

1 cup unsweetened vanilla almond milk

1 cup frozen strawberries

1 cup baby spinach

1 fresh or frozen banana

¾ cup plain low-fat Greek yogurt

1 tablespoon hemp seeds

In a blender, combine all the ingredients and blend until the desired consistency is achieved. Add more liquid as needed. Serve immediately.

Per serving:

Calories: 201; Total fat: 5g; Sodium: 131mg; Cholesterol: 6mg; Total carbs: 32g; Fiber: 5g; Sugar: 20g; Protein: 8g

Cherry Charlie Checker

Anti-Inflammatory, Brain Health, Heart Health

SERVES 2

My niece Charlie loves all food but this smoothie makes her twist and shout. The dark blues and reds from the mingling of fruits in this smoothie signify just how nutrient- and antioxidant-rich this blend is, and the high protein content of the yogurt and chia seeds provide a thick, creamy texture that will keep you full and satisfied.

1 cup skim milk

1 cup frozen blueberries

1 fresh or frozen banana

¾ cup plain low-fat Greek

yogurt ½ cup frozen cherries

½ cup frozen strawberries

1 tablespoon chia seeds

In a blender, combine all the ingredients and blend until the desired consistency is achieved. Add more liquid as needed. Serve immediately.

Per serving:

Calories: 265; Total fat: 5g; Sodium: 133mg; Cholesterol: 8mg; Total carbs: 48g; Fiber: 8g; Sugar: 32g; Protein: 12g

Bear's Choice

Anti-Inflammatory, Heart Health, Immune Boost

SERVES 2

Early in our relationship, I gave my husband the nickname Bear because he looks like a cute brown bear and he steals and eats all my berries from the refrigerator like a bear foraging in the woods. He also happens to idolize the Grateful Dead, so the whole bear theme just naturally stuck. This recipe is obviously Bear-tested and approved.

1 cup unsweetened vanilla almond milk

1 cup baby spinach

1 fresh or frozen banana

¾ cup frozen blackberries

¾ cup frozen raspberries

¾ cup plain low-fat Greek yogurt

1 tablespoon hemp seeds

In a blender, combine all the ingredients and blend until the desired consistency is achieved. Add more liquid as needed. Serve immediately.

Bonus Boost:

The vitamin C content of the fruits in this smoothie will enhance iron absorption from the spinach and these fruits also provide a fiber- and potassium-rich blend of nutrients.

Per serving:

Calories: 224; Total fat: 6g; Sodium: 134mg; Cholesterol: 5mg; Total carbs: 37g; Fiber: 9g; Sugar: 24g; Protein: 9g

Rosy-Red Robin

Anti-Inflammatory, Heart Health

SERVES 2

My friend Robin is a dietitian and personal trainer who is always inspiring me to find ways to use interesting superfood ingredients in my meals. Plus, she always wears this great shade of rosy-red lipstick that I should inquire about the next time I see her. This smoothie combines the bright colors and tart flavors of red fruits, particularly cranberries and raspberries, with the sweetness of banana and low-sugar vanilla yogurt to balance out the flavors.

1 cup unsweetened vanilla almond milk

1 cup frozen raspberries

1 fresh or frozen banana

¾ cup Siggi's vanilla yogurt

½ cup frozen strawberries

½ cup frozen cranberries 1

tablespoon chia seeds

In a blender, combine all the ingredients and blend until the desired consistency is achieved. Add more liquid as needed. Serve immediately.

Bonus Boost:

Cranberries are high in antioxidants, fiber, and unique plant compounds called polyphenols but are rarely eaten raw due to their flavor, so this recipe is a way to incorporate their nutritious benefits into your diet.

Per serving:

Calories: 239; Total fat: 7g; Sodium: 112mg; Cholesterol: 12mg; Total

carbs: 38g; Fiber: 11g; Sugar: 20g; Protein: 7g

Pom Dot Com

Anti-Inflammatory, Brain Health, Heart Health, Immune Boost

SERVES 2

The seeds or arils are the edible part of a pomegranate. You can buy them separately in most markets and they contain tons of antioxidants and special plant compounds unique to this fruit. To reap all their powerful nutrition benefits, you can use them in a smoothie but make sure to blend the tough seeds longer so they incorporate into the mix. Pomegranate juice is also an option if you can't find the seeds. A splash of orange juice boosts the sweetness in this blend.

1 cup unsweetened vanilla coconut milk

1 cup frozen blackberries

1 cup frozen raspberries

1 cup baby spinach

1 cup plain coconut yogurt

¼ cup orange juice

¼ cup pomegranate arils

1 tablespoon chia seeds

In a blender, combine all the ingredients and blend until the desired consistency is achieved. Add more liquid as needed and blend longer to make sure the pomegranate arils are incorporated. Serve immediately.

Per serving:

Calories: 263; Total fat: 9g; Sodium: 126mg; Cholesterol: 0mg; Total carbs: 41g; Fiber: 13g; Sugar: 26g; Protein: 9g

Rainbow Bright

Anti-Inflammatory, Brain Health, Digestive Health, Heart Health, Immune Boost

SERVES 2

This colorful recipe blends sweeter fruits in a frozen tropical mix with pomegranate arils to balance out the flavors so no extra juice is needed. The extra antioxidant punch from the arils provides a bright addition to your typical smoothie recipe.

1 cup unsweetened vanilla almond milk

1 cup frozen strawberries

1 cup frozen tropical fruit mix

1 cup plain low-fat Greek yogurt

¼ cup pomegranate arils

1 tablespoon hemp seeds

In a blender, combine all the ingredients and blend until the desired consistency is achieved. Add more liquid as needed, and blend longer to make sure the pomegranate arils are incorporated. Serve immediately.

Per serving:

Calories: 220; Total fat: 6g; Sodium: 142mg; Cholesterol: 7mg; Total carbs: 34g; Fiber: 6g; Sugar: 24g; Protein: 10g

The Three Bears

Anti-Inflammatory, Heart Health, Immune Boost

SERVES 2

This heart-healthy blend tastes like oatmeal in a cup but better! No bear will leave the cottage growling and hungry after drinking this mix of ingredients, which combines filling, soluble fiber–rich oats and fruits with high-protein Greek yogurt and chia seeds.

1½ cups frozen strawberries

1 cup unsweetened oat milk

1 fresh or frozen banana

¾ cup plain low-fat Greek yogurt

½ cup rolled oats or oat flour

1 tablespoon chia seeds

In a blender, combine all the ingredients and blend until the desired consistency is achieved. Add more liquid as needed. Serve immediately.

Per serving:

Calories: 420; Total fat: 7g; Sodium: 74mg; Cholesterol: 6mg; Total carbs: 79g; Fiber: 14g; Sugar: 30g; Protein: 15g

Tropical Storm Theo

Anti-Inflammatory, Digestive Health, Heart Health

SERVES 2

I love buying ready-to-use unsweetened frozen fruit blends with unique ingredients for a lightning-quick smoothie option. The only thing stormier and more delicious than this blend is the two-year-old it was named after.

1½ cups frozen papaya blend (papaya, mango, strawberry, pineapple)

1 cup unsweetened coconut milk

1 fresh or frozen banana

¾ cup plain coconut yogurt

1 tablespoon hemp seeds

In a blender, combine all the ingredients and blend until the desired consistency is achieved. Add more liquid as needed. Serve immediately.

Bonus Boost:

Papaya is rich in vitamins A and C, which is great for skin and ocular health.

Per serving:

Calories: 203; Total fat: 7g; Sodium: 108mg; Cholesterol: 0mg; Total carbs: 31g; Fiber: 4g; Sugar: 21g; Protein: 6g

Nutty Nittany Lion

Brain Health, Heart Health

SERVES 2

This blend of heart-healthy protein and fat from nuts, seeds, and yogurt is a far cry from the junky college food I ate during my years at my alma mater, Penn State (Go, Nittany Lions!). I could have used this snack instead of pizza at 2 a.m.!

2 fresh or frozen bananas

1 cup unsweetened almond milk

1 cup baby spinach

¾ cup plain low-fat Greek

yogurt 4 ice cubes

1 tablespoon chia seeds

1 tablespoon almond butter

In a blender, combine all the ingredients and blend until the desired consistency is achieved. Add more liquid as needed. Serve immediately.

Bonus Boost:

Nuts are a great source of vitamin E, magnesium, and selenium for heart and bone health, are naturally low in carbohydrates, and are high in fat for blood sugar maintenance.

Per serving:

Calories: 273; Total fat: 10g; Sodium: 131mg; Cholesterol: 6mg; Total carbs: 39g; Fiber: 7g; Sugar: 23g; Protein: 10g

Alf's Apple Pie

Anti-Inflammatory, Heart Health

SERVES 2

If an apple a day really keeps the doctor away, try this smoothie for a nutritious variation on apple pie that will boost your immunity and keep you healthy in any season. Apples are a great source of fiber, vitamins, and minerals, and I recommend blending them up with the skin on to reap the most benefits. Although the show Alf with the furry alien was one of my childhood favorites, this smoothie was also named for one of my favorite families, the Alfs, who let me come over and test green smoothies on their kids.

1 cup unsweetened oat milk

1 cup chopped apple

1 fresh or frozen banana

¾ cup Siggi's whole-milk vanilla

yogurt ½ cup rolled oats or oat flour

Pinch ground cinnamon

In a blender, combine all the ingredients and blend until the desired consistency is achieved. Add more liquid as needed. Serve immediately.

Per serving:

Calories: 349; Total fat: 8g; Sodium: 49mg; Cholesterol: 12mg; Total carbs: 65g; Fiber: 8g; Sugar: 26g; Protein: 12g

Strawberry Summer 365

Anti-Inflammatory, Digestive Health, Heart Health, Immune Boost

SERVES 2

Summer can be served all year long with this peachy-keen smoothie full of summer fruits. The benefit of buying frozen fruit is that you can find most seasonal fruits, like peaches and berries, all year long.

1 cup unsweetened vanilla almond milk
1 cup frozen mixed berries
1 cup frozen peaches
1 cup baby spinach
¾ cup Siggi's whole-milk vanilla yogurt ½ cup water
1 tablespoon chia seeds

In a blender, combine all the ingredients and blend until the desired consistency is achieved. Add more liquid as needed. Serve immediately.

Per serving:
Calories: 171; Total fat: 7g; Sodium: 128mg; Cholesterol: 12mg; Total carbs: 23g; Fiber: 6g; Sugar: 16g; Protein: 6g

The Pretty Peach

Anti-Inflammatory, Heart Health, Immune Boost

SERVES 2

This colorful and tasty mix blends summer fruits with high-protein Greek yogurt for a refreshing smoothie any time of the day. It is almost as pretty as my friend Jaclyn, aka Peaches.

1 cup unsweetened vanilla almond milk
1 cup frozen peaches
1 cup frozen strawberries
1 cup baby spinach
¾ cup plain low-fat Greek
yogurt ½ cup frozen raspberries
1 tablespoon hemp seeds

In a blender, combine all the ingredients and blend until the desired consistency is achieved. Add more liquid as needed. Serve immediately.

Bonus Boost:

The vitamin C in the fruit will increase the absorption of iron from the spinach for a nutrient-rich winning combo.

Per serving:

Calories: 199; Total fat: 6g; Sodium: 142mg; Cholesterol: 6mg; Total carbs: 30g; Fiber: 7g; Sugar: 21g; Protein: 8g

Raspberry Rocks

Anti-Inflammatory, Heart Health, Immune Boost

SERVES 2

Turn on the kitchen tunes, break out the blender, and rock out with this red raspberry blend full of fiber and nutrients. With just a few staple ingredients that you probably have on hand, this classic tangy mix is a no-brainer for any meal or snack.

1 cup unsweetened vanilla almond milk

1 cup frozen raspberries

1 fresh or frozen banana

¾ cup plain low-fat Greek

yogurt 1 cup baby spinach

1 tablespoon hemp seeds

In a blender, combine all the ingredients and blend until the desired consistency is achieved. Add more liquid as needed. Serve immediately.

Bonus Boost:

Berries are naturally low in sugar and full of fiber, and banana and spinach add potassium to keep your ticker rockin' and rollin'.

Per serving:

Calories: 197; Total fat: 6g; Sodium: 132mg; Cholesterol: 6mg; Total carbs: 31g; Fiber: 7g; Sugar: 18g; Protein: 8g

Wholly Melon

Anti-Inflammatory, Brain Health, Digestive Health, Immune Boost

SERVES 2

Move over, berries, the melons are taking over this smoothie. Melons and bananas are full of water and important nutrients like folate, vitamin C, and potassium, and the addition of coconut yogurt and coconut milk provides even more hydration. Wholly melon, you're going to feel refreshed after this one!

1 cup unsweetened coconut milk

1 cup plain coconut yogurt

1 cup honeydew

1 cup cantaloupe

1 fresh or frozen banana

4 ice cubes

1 tablespoon chia seeds

In a blender, combine all the ingredients and blend until the desired consistency is achieved. Add more liquid as needed. Serve immediately.

Per serving:

Calories: 244; Total fat: 8g; Sodium: 154mg; Cholesterol: 0mg; Total carbs: 38g; Fiber: 6g; Sugar: 29g; Protein: 8g

Sweet Tater

Heart Health, Immune Boost

SERVES 2

I am not welcome at any holiday feast without my famous sweet potato pies full of butter, cream, and sugar, so naturally I had to "healthify" this decadent treat. This smoothie tastes just like my dreamy pies in a cup but without the unwanted calories.

1 cup unsweetened vanilla almond milk

1 cup cooked sweet potato

1 cup frozen mango

1 cup baby spinach (optional)

Dash ground cinnamon

Dash ground nutmeg

Dash ground ginger

In a blender, combine all the ingredients and blend until the desired consistency is achieved. Add more liquid as needed. Serve immediately.

Bonus Boost:

Sweet potatoes are a great source of complex carbs and antioxidant-rich beta-carotene, and the nut milk and spices mimic the rich ingredients in my pies so you stay full and happy just like after a holiday meal (without the need to unbutton your pants).

Per serving:

Calories: 195; Total fat: 2g; Sodium: 121mg; Cholesterol: 0mg; Total carbs: 42g; Fiber: 6g; Sugar: 22g; Protein: 3g

Cherry Michele Chanel

Anti-Inflammatory, Digestive Health, Heart Health

SERVES 2

This deep-red smoothie sounds and looks fancy but it is as simple and genuine as my friend Michele. Frozen cherries come without the pits and are ready to blend, and they're bursting with antioxidants and natural sweetness. The optional sprinkle of chocolate on top could change the name to Coco Chanel, but we'll save that for the next smoothie book.

2 cups frozen dark cherries

1 cup unsweetened vanilla almond milk

¾ cup plain low-fat Greek yogurt

1 tablespoon hemp seeds

Mini dark chocolate chips, for sprinkling on top (optional)

In a blender, combine all the ingredients (except the optional chocolate chips) and blend until the desired consistency is achieved. Add more liquid as needed. Sprinkle the chocolate chips (if using) on top and serve immediately.

Per serving:

Calories: 175; Total fat: 6g; Sodium: 139mg; Cholesterol: 6mg; Total carbs: 25g; Fiber: 3g; Sugar: 22g; Protein: 8g

Macho Green Matcha

Anti-Inflammatory, Brain Health, Heart Health, Immune Boost

SERVES 2

Green tea powder, aka matcha powder, will not only make you feel mucho energized from a kick of caffeine, but it will give your body a dose of heart-healthy antioxidants. When this bitter powder is blended with the natural sweetness from banana, mango, and coconut, the balance is a work of matcha-ral beauty.

1 cup unsweetened coconut milk

1 cup frozen mango

1 cup baby spinach

1 fresh or frozen banana

¾ cup plain coconut yogurt

1 tablespoon chia seeds

2 teaspoons matcha powder

In a blender, combine all the ingredients and blend until the desired consistency is achieved. Add more liquid as needed. Serve immediately.

Per serving:

Calories: 224; Total fat: 7g; Sodium: 134mg; Cholesterol: 0mg; Total carbs: 36g; Fiber: 7g; Sugar: 24g; Protein: 7g

The Vitamin C Note

Anti-Inflammatory, Digestive Health, Heart Health, Immune Boost

SERVES 2

Wait and see how this vitamin C–rich blend will give you that boost of immunity and make you feel like a stack of C-notes. The trio of fruit, seeds, and yogurt not only tastes Cen-sational but might also even give you a nice glow.

1 cup unsweetened vanilla almond milk

1 cup cantaloupe

1 cup frozen strawberries

¾ cup plain low-fat Greek

yogurt 1 clementine

1 tablespoon chia seeds

In a blender, combine all the ingredients and blend until the desired consistency is achieved. Add more liquid as needed. Serve immediately.

Per serving:

Calories: 199; Total fat: 5g; Sodium: 148mg; Cholesterol: 6mg; Total carbs: 32g; Fiber: 7g; Sugar: 23g; Protein: 8g

Eddie B's Monday-Morning Doubles

Anti-Inflammatory, Heart Health

SERVES 2

Ace it like Grandpa Eddie does when you double down on this coffee drink with two sources of caffeinated goodness to add an energizing kick to your game. The coffee flour, made from dried coffee cherry husks, is from Trader Joe's and is not necessary but just a tiny amount provides a hearty 6 grams of fiber! Although this blend tastes like an indulgent coffee shop frappuccino, it's a healthy choice with tons of nutrient-rich fruits and veggies and a dose of satiating protein from Greek yogurt. The advantage is in your court!

1 cup frozen strawberries

1 cup kale

1 fresh or frozen banana

¾ cup plain low-fat Greek yogurt

½ cup unsweetened vanilla almond milk

½ cup coffee

1 teaspoon coffee powder

In a blender, combine all the ingredients and blend until the desired consistency is achieved. Add more liquid as needed. Serve immediately.

Per serving:

Calories: 153; Total fat: 2g; Sodium: 109mg; Cholesterol: 6mg; Total carbs: 28g; Fiber: 4g; Sugar: 17g; Protein: 7g

Zurprise!

Anti-Inflammatory, Heart Health, Immune Boost

SERVES 2

There's a zecret zurprise in this smoothie that you would never detect if you didn't read the ingredients. I know you're reading them now, so let's discuss zucchini. Its neutral taste and nutritious profile make it a perfect addition to any smoothie. You can buy it sliced or spiralized in the freezer so it goes straight into the blender with the other ingredients. You will feel like you got whisked off to an island zurprise getaway.

1 cup unsweetened vanilla almond milk

1 cup frozen tropical fruit mix

1 cup frozen zucchini spirals

1 fresh or frozen banana

¾ cup plain low-fat Greek yogurt

In a blender, combine all the ingredients and blend until the desired consistency is achieved. Add more liquid as needed. Serve immediately.

Per serving:

Calories: 200; Total fat: 4g; Sodium: 138mg; Cholesterol: 6mg; Total carbs: 37g; Fiber: 6g; Sugar: 28g; Protein: 8g

Banana Buddhaberry

Anti-Inflammatory, Brain Health, Heart Health, Immune Boost

SERVES 2

You'll be smiling like a buddha when you get a taste of this banana berrylicious blend of iron- and fiber-rich ingredients. The yogurt and hemp seeds provide protein and heart-healthy fat to turn that hungry frown upside down.

1 cup unsweetened vanilla almond milk

1 cup frozen raspberries

1 cup baby spinach

1 fresh or frozen banana

¾ cup plain low-fat Greek yogurt

1 tablespoon hemp seeds

In a blender, combine all the ingredients and blend until the desired consistency is achieved. Add more liquid as needed. Serve immediately.

Per serving:

Calories: 198; Total fat: 6g; Sodium: 141mg; Cholesterol: 6mg; Total carbs: 30g; Fiber: 7g; Sugar: 18g; Protein: 8g

Naked Nut-trition

Anti-Inflammatory, Brain Health, Heart Health

SERVES 2

My online persona is Get Naked Nutrition, which teaches you how to incorporate more naked foods (fruits, veggies, and other real foods without labels) into your diet so you feel better naked. A win-win! Like all the smoothies in this book, this one uses naked ingredients, including all-mighty nuts that naturally provide all three macronutrients your body needs. It's totally nuts how this combo of carbs, protein, and fat coupled with bananas and protein-rich yogurt will keep you so satisfied.

2 fresh or frozen bananas

1 cup unsweetened vanilla almond milk

1 cup baby spinach

¾ cup plain low-fat Greek

yogurt 4 large ice cubes

1 tablespoon almond butter

1 tablespoon peanut butter

In a blender, combine all the ingredients and blend until the desired consistency is achieved. Add more liquid as needed. Serve immediately.

Per serving:

Calories: 285; Total fat: 12g; Sodium: 182mg; Cholesterol: 6mg; Total carbs: 38g; Fiber: 5g; Sugar: 22g; Protein: 11g

The Sammer Jammer

Anti-Inflammatory, Heart Health, Immune Boost

SERVES 2

This smoothie is a Burak household favorite, especially for my seven-year-old son Sam, aka Sammer. He asks for this combo on a daily basis and if he doesn't detect the antioxidant- and fiber-rich spinach and chia seeds in here, you won't either.

1 cup unsweetened vanilla almond milk

1 cup frozen raspberries

1 cup frozen mango

1 cup baby spinach

¾ cup plain low-fat Greek

yogurt 1 tablespoon chia seeds

In a blender, combine all the ingredients and blend until the desired consistency is achieved. Add more liquid as needed. Serve immediately.

Per serving:

Calories: 202; Total fat: 6g; Sodium: 142mg; Cholesterol: 6mg; Total carbs: 31g; Fiber: 9g; Sugar: 21g; Protein: 8g

It's Cocopletely Bananas

Anti-Inflammatory, Brain Health

SERVES 2

You will go totally bananas for this coconutty chocolate combo that will take care of any sweet hankering. Coconut is mostly fat, specifically MCTs or medium-chain triglycerides. Your body metabolizes these fats differently than others and is able to quickly use them for energy so you will feel cocopletely satisfied.

1 cup unsweetened vanilla almond milk

1 cup frozen coconut pieces

1 cup baby spinach

1 fresh or frozen banana

4 tablespoons chocolate hemp protein powder

1 tablespoon cacao powder

In a blender, combine all the ingredients and blend until the desired consistency is achieved. Add more liquid as needed. Serve immediately.

Per serving:

Calories: 231; Total fat: 12g; Sodium: 113mg; Cholesterol: 2mg; Total carbs: 21g; Fiber: 6g; Sugar: 11g; Protein: 12g

Patty Papaya

Anti-Inflammatory, Brain Health, Digestive Health, Heart Health, Immune Boost

SERVES 2

This colorful smoothie is a nod to Patty, my hairdresser, who has a different shade of red or orange hair every time I see her. She makes sure my grays are covered every month, so she certainly deserves a smoothie with her name on it. Papaya is the star in this combo, which is a great source of carotenoids, particularly lycopene, a powerful disease-fighting antioxidant.

1 cup unsweetened coconut milk

1 cup frozen tropical fruit mix

1 cup frozen papaya

1 cup baby spinach

¾ cup plain coconut yogurt

1 tablespoon chia seeds

In a blender, combine all the ingredients and blend until the desired consistency is achieved. Add more liquid as needed. Serve immediately.

Per serving:

Calories: 198; Total fat: 7g; Sodium: 127mg; Cholesterol: 0mg; Total carbs: 29g; Fiber: 7g; Sugar: 21g; Protein: 7g

Minty Makeover

SERVES 2

Make over your typical fruit smoothie with the addition of invigorating mint leaves. This blend combines plant-based yogurt, milk, and seeds for a nutrient-dense flavor profile. Mint is great for digestion and inflammation, plus it doesn't hurt to freshen up your kisser at the same time.

1 cup unsweetened vanilla almond milk

1 cup frozen strawberries

1 cup frozen mango

¾ cup plain coconut yogurt

Few fresh mint leaves

1 tablespoon hemp seeds

In a blender, combine all the ingredients and blend until the desired consistency is achieved. Add more liquid as needed. Serve immediately.

Per serving:

Calories: 193; Total fat: 7g; Sodium: 121mg; Cholesterol: 0mg; Total carbs: 28g; Fiber: 5g; Sugar: 22g; Protein: 6g

Jerry's Purple Jam

Anti-Inflammatory, Brain Health, Heart Health, Immune Boost

SERVES 2

Blueberries and blackberries are to superfoods as Jerry was to jamming, so this smoothie is a musical masterpiece. Don't confuse hemp seeds with the mind-altering parts of the plant that you may see at a Dead show. This type of hemp is a nutritionist's dream—rich in protein, fiber, and heart-healthy fats. Within your first few sips of this drink, there will be nothing left to do but smile, smile, smile.

1 cup unsweetened hemp milk

1 cup frozen blueberries

1 cup frozen blackberries

¾ cup vanilla or plain low-fat Greek

yogurt 1 tablespoon hemp seeds

In a blender, combine all the ingredients and blend until the desired consistency is achieved. Add more liquid as needed. Serve immediately.

Per serving:

Calories: 194; Total fat: 6g; Sodium: 139mg; Cholesterol: 6mg; Total carbs: 29g; Fiber: 7g; Sugar: 21g; Protein: 7g

The Baked Big Apple

Anti-Inflammatory, Digestive Health, Heart Health

SERVES 2

Start spreadin' the news that it only takes minutes to blend up a treat that tastes like a baked apple pie but without the sugar high. Soluble fiber–rich apples and pears are blended with vanilla yogurt for a satisfying combo that will help keep your gut healthy and happy.

1 cup unsweetened vanilla almond milk

1 cup apple chunks

1 cup pear chunks

¾ cup Siggi's whole-milk vanilla

yogurt 1 tablespoon hemp seeds

1 tablespoon rolled oats

Dash ground cinnamon

In a blender, combine all the ingredients and blend until the desired consistency is achieved. Add more liquid as needed. Serve immediately.

Per serving:

Calories: 196; Total fat: 7g; Sodium: 118mg; Cholesterol: 12mg; Total carbs: 29g; Fiber: 5g; Sugar: 19g; Protein: 6g

Classic Creamsicle

Heart Health

SERVES 2

The classic creamsicle is back and the only thing it lacks is added sugar. A blend of vitamin C–rich orange fruits with filling yogurt and chia seeds tastes like such a treat that it will make you forget all about the old-school ice-pop version you loved as a kid.

1 cup unsweetened vanilla almond milk

1 cup frozen mango

2 mandarin oranges

¾ cup Siggi's whole-milk vanilla

yogurt 1 tablespoon chia seeds

1 teaspoon vanilla extract

In a blender, combine all the ingredients and blend until the desired consistency is achieved. Add more liquid as needed. Serve immediately.

Per serving:

Calories: 201; Total fat: 7g; Sodium: 119mg; Cholesterol: 12mg; Total carbs: 30g; Fiber: 5g; Sugar: 24g; Protein: 6g

Metabolic Machine

Anti-Inflammatory, Brain Health, Immune Boost

SERVES 2

Give your metabolism a boost with this blend of fiber, protein, and fat from bananas, almond butter, and seeds. This key combo controls your blood sugar and keeps your engine working at peak so you stay full and satisfied.

2 fresh or frozen bananas

1 cup unsweetened vanilla almond milk

1 cup baby spinach

¾ cup plain low-fat Greek yogurt

1 tablespoon almond butter

1 tablespoon chia/hemp/flaxseed

mix Dash ground cinnamon

In a blender, combine all the ingredients and blend until the desired consistency is achieved. Add more liquid as needed. Serve immediately.

Bonus Boost:

Cinnamon adds sweetness without sugar and contains powerful antioxidants and compounds that can help reduce insulin resistance, which is excellent for blood sugar maintenance.

Per serving:

Calories: 276; Total fat: 10g; Sodium: 139mg; Cholesterol: 6mg; Total carbs: 39g; Fiber: 7g; Sugar: 23g; Protein: 10g

Ahhh-mazing Acai

Anti-Inflammatory, Brain Health, Digestive Health, Heart Health, Immune Boost

SERVES 2

Acai is an antioxidant-rich fruit from the rain forest that provides a slew of vitamins and minerals. You may have seen it in its bowl form before. An acai bowl is really just a smoothie in a bowl so if pouring this blend straight from the blender into a bowl and adding toppings like fresh fruit and coconut flakes makes you happy, be my guest!

1 cup unsweetened hemp milk

1 fresh or frozen banana

¾ cup plain coconut

yogurt 1 cup baby spinach

1 (3.5-ounce) packet frozen acai

1 tablespoon hemp seeds

In a blender, combine all the ingredients and blend until the desired consistency is achieved. Add more liquid as needed. Serve immediately.

Bonus Boost:

Although acai berries are a fruit, they are also a great source of omega-3 heart-healthy fats! Plus, they're full of fiber to keep your digestive system nice and regular.

Per serving:

Calories: 213; Total fat: 11g; Sodium: 131mg; Cholesterol: 0mg; Total carbs: 22g; Fiber: 3g; Sugar: 21g; Protein: 7g

Not Yo Mama's Matcha

Anti-Inflammatory, Digestive Health, Immune Boost

SERVES 2

Move over, tired mamas, a new matcha is in town. Antioxidant-rich green tea powder, or matcha, is blended with sweet, nutritious fruits and heart-healthy hemp for a boost of energy to get you through those long days.

1 cup unsweetened almond milk

1 cup frozen pineapple

1 fresh or frozen banana

¾ cup plain coconut yogurt

1 tablespoon hemp seeds

2 teaspoons matcha powder

In a blender, combine all the ingredients and blend until the desired consistency is achieved. Add more liquid as needed. Serve immediately.

Per serving:

Calories: 197; Total fat: 7g; Sodium: 120mg; Cholesterol: 0mg; Total carbs: 30g; Fiber: 4g; Sugar: 21g; Protein: 6g

Keri's Berries

Anti-Inflammatory, Brain Health, Heart Health, Immune Boost

SERVES 2

This smoothie is a berrylicious nod to my amazing nutrition mentor Keri, who not only makes a mean smoothie but is also a superstar in the world of nutrition—just like this trio of berries that are full of fiber and antioxidants.

1 cup unsweetened vanilla almond milk

1 cup strawberries

¾ cup plain low-fat Greek

yogurt ½ cup raspberries

½ cup blueberries

1 tablespoon chia/flax/hemp seed mix

1 teaspoon greens powder (optional)

In a blender, combine all the ingredients and blend until the desired consistency is achieved. Add more liquid as needed. Serve immediately.

Bonus Boost:

When berries are blended with optional greens powder and a seed mix, the nutrient profile of this drink gets an A+.

Per serving:

Calories: 178; Total fat: 5g; Sodium: 142mg; Cholesterol: 6mg; Total carbs: 24g; Fiber: 7g; Sugar: 16g; Protein: 8g

Eye of the Pumpkin

Anti-Inflammatory, Digestive Health, Heart Health, Immune Boost

SERVES 2

When the holiday season comes to an end, pumpkins tend to take a backseat to other orange, beta-carotene-rich gems. But the truth is, canned pumpkin is one of the best nutritional bangs for your buck. A little dollop of pumpkin adds a nutritious punch to smoothies and other recipes.

1 cup pure canned pumpkin

1 cup kale

1 fresh or frozen banana

¾ cup Siggi's whole-milk vanilla

yogurt ½ cup unsweetened hemp milk

1 tablespoon hemp seeds

Dash ground cinnamon

In a blender, combine all the ingredients and blend until the desired consistency is achieved. Add more liquid as needed. Serve immediately.

Per serving:
Calories: 210; Total fat: 7g; Sodium: 81mg; Cholesterol: 17mg; Total carbs: 32g; Fiber: 6g; Sugar: 19g; Protein: 8g

JP's Green Garden

Anti-Inflammatory, Brain Health, Digestive Health, Heart Health

SERVES 2

This recipe is inspired by a wonderful Mexican chef whom I met on vacation while writing this book. All his dishes contain ingredients grown in the restaurant's garden and I was reminded how some veggies and herbs not only provide smoothies with unique flavor and nutrient profiles but are also an amazing cure for too much tequila the night before.

1 cup unsweetened coconut milk

1 cup frozen mango

1 cup frozen pineapple

¾ cup plain coconut yogurt

½ cup peeled cucumber

1 teaspoon spirulina

Few fresh mint leaves

In a blender, combine all the ingredients and blend until the desired consistency is achieved. Add more liquid as needed. Serve immediately.

Per serving:

Calories: 175; Total fat: 5g; Sodium: 132mg; Cholesterol: 0mg; Total carbs: 29g; Fiber: 3g; Sugar: 26g; Protein: 6g

Al's Iced Hazelnut

Brain Health, Heart Health

SERVES 2

Just like my best friend Allison, who cannot function unless she drinks two hazelnut iced coffees a day, this peanut-buttery banana blend will never let you down. It is full of satiating protein, fiber, and heart-healthy fat, unlike traditional calorie-bomb milkshakes. A hint of hazelnut or plain coffee is the icing on the cake.

2 fresh or frozen bananas

1 cup kale

¾ cup plain low-fat Greek yogurt

½ cup leftover hazelnut or regular coffee

½ cup unsweetened vanilla almond

milk 1 tablespoon hemp seeds

1 tablespoon peanut butter

In a blender, combine all the ingredients and blend until the desired consistency is achieved. Add more liquid as needed. Serve immediately.

Per serving:

Calories: 240; Total fat: 10g; Sodium: 132mg; Cholesterol: 6mg; Total carbs: 34g; Fiber: 4g; Sugar: 20g; Protein: 9g

Workout Wonder

Anti-Inflammatory, Heart Health, Immune Boost

SERVES 2

Don't let this cute name fool you: You can blend up this mix of nutritious ingredients anytime, whether you just worked out or not, to provide a fiber- and protein-packed smoothie option. If you want to experiment with protein powders, I recommend trying single-serving packs first (instead of giant tubs) to test your taste preferences. Feel free to sub in yogurt instead.

1 cup unsweetened vanilla almond milk

1 cup frozen blueberries

1 cup baby spinach

1 fresh or frozen banana

2 scoops plain whey, pea, or hemp protein powder

1 tablespoon almond butter

1 tablespoon chia seeds

In a blender, combine all the ingredients and blend until the desired consistency is achieved. Add more liquid as needed. Serve immediately.

Per serving:

Calories: 303; Total fat: 9g; Sodium: 197mg; Cholesterol: 3mg; Total carbs: 37g; Fiber: 8g; Sugar: 16g; Protein: 21g

Cup of Joe Schmo

Anti-Inflammatory, Digestive Health, Heart Health

SERVES 2

This smoothie is not your average cup of joe. Spice it up by adding espresso powder and leftover coffee to sweet, nutritious fruits for a twist on your classic frozen coffee blend. Feel free to sub in your choice of yogurt for the protein powder.

1 cup frozen cherries

1 cup kale

½ fresh or frozen banana

½ cup frozen raspberries

½ cup leftover coffee

½ cup unsweetened vanilla almond milk

2 scoops plain whey, hemp, or pea protein powder

1 teaspoon espresso or coffee powder (optional)

In a blender, combine all the ingredients and blend until the desired consistency is achieved. Add more liquid as needed. Serve immediately.

Per serving:

Calories: 185; Total fat: 2g; Sodium: 150mg; Cholesterol: 3mg; Total carbs: 25g; Fiber: 5g; Sugar: 10g; Protein: 19g

Grateful Green

Anti-Inflammatory, Brain Health, Heart Health

SERVES 2

You'll be grateful that you gave green a chance once you taste this smoothie bursting with nutrients from a variety of fruits and veggies. If you don't have one of the leafy green ingredients, feel free to double up on the other.

1 cup unsweetened coconut milk

1 cup frozen tropical fruit mix

1 cup baby spinach

1 cup kale

1 fresh or frozen banana

¾ cup plain coconut yogurt

¼ cup frozen avocado or ¼ fresh avocado

In a blender, combine all the ingredients and blend until the desired consistency is achieved. Add more liquid as needed. Serve immediately.

Per serving:

Calories: 220; Total fat: 8g; Sodium: 135mg; Cholesterol: 0mg; Total carbs: 34g; Fiber: 7g; Sugar: 23g; Protein: 7g

The Bold Lip

Heart Health, Immune Boost

SERVES 2

Pucker up, because you've found your new favorite immunity-boosting diet accessory. This ripe-red smoothie is bursting with vitamin C–rich fruits and protein-filled yogurt and chia seeds for a tasty, bold treat that tastes so good when it hits your lips.

1 cup unsweetened almond milk

1 cup frozen cherries

1 cup baby spinach

¾ cup plain low-fat Greek

yogurt 1 mandarin orange

½ cup frozen strawberries

1 tablespoon chia seeds

In a blender, combine all the ingredients and blend until the desired consistency is achieved. Add more liquid as needed. Serve immediately.

Per serving:

Calories: 190; Total fat: 5g; Sodium: 145mg; Cholesterol: 6mg; Total carbs: 29g; Fiber: 6g; Sugar: 21g; Protein: 8g

The Waterlemon

Anti-Inflammatory, Brain Health, Digestive Health

SERVES 2

Lemonade is usually laden with added sugar but this take on a frosty watermelon lemonade contains only natural sweetness from a hydrating mix of fruits with creamy coconut yogurt and coconut milk.

1 cup unsweetened coconut milk or water

1 cup watermelon

1 cup frozen mango

¾ cup plain coconut

yogurt Juice of ½ lemon

1 tablespoon hemp seeds

In a blender, combine all the ingredients and blend until the desired consistency is achieved. Add more liquid as needed. Serve immediately.

Per serving:

Calories: 157; Total fat: 6g; Sodium: 44mg; Cholesterol: 0mg; Total carbs: 24g; Fiber: 2g; Sugar: 20g; Protein: 5g

Hirsch's Kiss

Anti-Inflammatory, Brain Health, Immune Boost

SERVES 2

Kiss your sweet tooth goodbye with this nutritious version of a chocolate, peanut butter, coconut masterpiece that is bursting with hidden fiber and antioxidant-rich extras from cauliflower and hemp. If your taste buds are ready to party, this blend will not disappoint, just like my fun friends the Hirsches, from whom this smoothie takes its name.

1 cup unsweetened hemp milk

1 cup frozen coconut chunks

1 fresh or frozen banana

¾ cup plain low-fat Greek yogurt

½ cup frozen riced cauliflower

1 tablespoon peanut butter

1 tablespoon cacao powder

1 tablespoon hemp seeds

In a blender, combine all the ingredients and blend until the desired consistency is achieved. Add more liquid as needed. Serve immediately.

Per serving:

Calories: 338; Total fat: 18g; Sodium: 170mg; Cholesterol: 15mg; Total carbs: 35g; Fiber: 6g; Sugar: 23g; Protein: 14g

Wind Me Up

Anti-Inflammatory, Heart Health

SERVES 2

Wind up your week with this caffeinated blend of chocolatey, nutty goodness. Potassium- and fiber-rich fruits and spinach provide a dose of complex carbs, while hemp seeds and almond butter pump up the protein and heart-healthy fats to stabilize blood sugar and keep your engine revved up.

1 cup frozen blueberries

1 cup baby spinach or kale

1 fresh or frozen banana

½ cup leftover coffee

½ cup unsweetened vanilla almond

milk 1 tablespoon hemp seeds

1 tablespoon cacao powder

1 tablespoon almond butter

In a blender, combine all the ingredients and blend until the desired consistency is achieved. Add more liquid as needed. Serve immediately.

Per serving:

Calories: 176; Total fat: 8g; Sodium: 45mg; Cholesterol: 0mg; Total carbs: 24g; Fiber: 6g; Sugar: 12g; Protein: 5g

Salty Peanut Butter Pretzel

Anti-Inflammatory, Brain Health, Heart Health

SERVES 2

If you love the combo of sweet and salty like I do, then this blend has your name on it. There's nothing better than the taste and nutrition of merging bananas with peanut butter. But when you add in nutritional boosts of fiber, protein, and healthy fats from the zucchini, hemp, and Greek yogurt, your metabolism will thank you even more. Dashes of cinnamon and sea salt round out the flavors and provide additional antioxidants and minerals.

2 fresh or frozen bananas

1 cup unsweetened vanilla almond milk

¾ cup plain low-fat Greek

yogurt ½ cup frozen zucchini

1 tablespoon hemp seeds

1 tablespoon peanut

butter Dash sea salt

Dash ground cinnamon

In a blender, combine all the ingredients and blend until the desired consistency is achieved. Add more liquid as needed. Serve immediately.

Per serving:

Calories: 262; Total fat: 10g; Sodium: 232mg; Cholesterol: 6mg; Total carbs: 38g; Fiber: 5g; Sugar: 24g; Protein: 10g

Sabrina's Spicy A.M. Shake-Up

Anti-Inflammatory, Brain Health, Heart Health

SERVES 2

Shake up your early morning routine with the Queen Bee of invigorating smoothies. Aunt Sabrina has always been a morning person but even she needs a pick-me-up once in a while to get her through a long day of teaching her class. Small hits of ginger and cayenne pack a spicy punch that will kick up your regular fruit smoothie and possibly provide a temporary metabolic boost due to the slight thermogenic (heat-producing) effect of spicy food on your system. Some studies even indicate spicy foods keep you fuller longer. Bonus!

1 cup unsweetened coconut milk

1 cup frozen mango

1 cup baby spinach or kale

1 fresh or frozen banana

¾ cup plain coconut yogurt

1 tablespoon chia seeds

1 tablespoon fresh ginger or 2 teaspoons ground

ginger ¼ teaspoon ground cayenne

In a blender, combine all the ingredients and blend until the desired consistency is achieved. Add more liquid as needed. Serve immediately.

Per serving:

Calories: 220; Total fat: 7g; Sodium: 124mg; Cholesterol: 12mg; Total carbs: 35g; Fiber: 6g; Sugar: 25g; Protein: 6g

The Superfruit Edition

Anti-Inflammatory, Brain Health, Heart Health, Immune Boost

SERVES 2

Even if you can't pronounce acai (say it with me: ahh-sah-EE), I'm sure you've heard about its superfruit powers. Combined with antioxidant-rich blueberries and pineapple, acai provides the icing on the nutritious cake in this purple blend full of polyphenols, aka your body's disease-preventing bestie. Feel free to blend the chia and coconut up with the other ingredients, or pour the mixture into a bowl, sprinkle them on top, and grab a spoon!

1 cup unsweetened coconut milk

1 cup baby spinach or kale

¾ cup plain coconut yogurt

½ cup frozen blueberries ½
cup frozen pineapple

1 (3.5-ounce) packet frozen acai

1 tablespoon chia seeds

1 tablespoon unsweetened shredded coconut

In a blender, combine all the ingredients and blend until the desired consistency is achieved. Add more liquid as needed. Serve immediately.

Per serving:
Calories: 255; Total fat: 14g; Sodium: 121mg; Cholesterol: 0mg; Total carbs: 23g; Fiber: 7g; Sugar: 15g; Protein: 6g

Pop Pop's Parrothead Piña Colada

Anti-Inflammatory, Brain Health, Immune Boost

SERVES 2

Even though he doesn't travel to the tropics often, my dad still enjoys Jimmy Buffett music and piña coladas anytime. This mix of tropical fruits, nuts, and seeds is a tasty combo full of antioxidants and heart-healthy fats. Although it tastes like a traditional sugary vacation cocktail, there is zero added sugar. Sub in any nut or seed butter if you don't have macadamia and feel free to sprinkle some coconut on top.

1 cup unsweetened almond milk

1 cup frozen pineapple

¾ cup plain coconut yogurt

½ cup frozen coconut

½ cup frozen mango

1 tablespoon macadamia nut butter

1 tablespoon hemp seeds

1 tablespoon unsweetened shredded coconut

In a blender, combine all the ingredients and blend until the desired consistency is achieved. Add more liquid as needed. Serve immediately.

Per serving:

Calories: 270; Total fat: 15g; Sodium: 124mg; Cholesterol: 0mg; Total carbs: 27g; Fiber: 4g; Sugar: 21g; Protein: 7g

The GG (Great Green)

Digestive Health, Heart Health

SERVES 2

This great blend is the matriarch of green smoothies, just like Grandma AG is to our family. The sweet tropical fruits balance out the green nutritional superfoods avocado and spinach so you may not believe you're drinking a big cup of green goodness.

2 cups baby spinach

1 cup unsweetened vanilla almond milk

1 cup frozen pineapple

1 fresh or frozen banana

¾ cup plain coconut yogurt

¼ cup frozen avocado or ¼ fresh

avocado 1 tablespoon ground flax meal

In a blender, combine all the ingredients and blend until the desired consistency is achieved. Add more liquid as needed. Serve immediately.

Bonus Boost:

Vitamin C, potassium, and protective fats stand out in this mix to keep your skin glowing and your heart strong.

Per serving:

Calories: 251; Total fat: 10g; Sodium: 138mg; Cholesterol: 0mg; Total carbs: 35g; Fiber: 7g; Sugar: 22g; Protein: 7g

Mama's Milkshake

Anti-Inflammatory, Heart Health, Immune Boost

SERVES 2

Shake it up, mamas, because you deserve a healthy treat for your hard work. This blend may resemble a creamy diner milkshake but the nutritious fruit pair mixed with high-protein yogurt and a double dose of hemp will keep your blood sugar and hunger levels stable (so when the kids get home, there's less of a chance you will scream your head off). You can also sub in any plain protein powder with a dash of pure vanilla extract or skip it altogether.

1 cup unsweetened vanilla almond milk

1 cup frozen strawberries

1 fresh or frozen banana

¾ cup Siggi's whole-milk vanilla

yogurt 1 scoop vanilla hemp protein

powder 1 tablespoon hemp seeds

In a blender, combine all the ingredients and blend until the desired consistency is achieved. Add more liquid as needed. Serve immediately.

Per serving:

Calories: 275; Total fat: 8g; Sodium: 199mg; Cholesterol: 12mg; Total carbs: 39g; Fiber: 5g; Sugar: 27g; Protein: 16g

Banana Splitz

Anti-Inflammatory, Heart Health, Immune Boost

SERVES 2

This grown-up version of your childhood favorite is so healthy and low cal that there is no need to split it between friends. Instead of the cherries on top, you can blend them right in to boost the antioxidant and anti-inflammatory properties of this combo. Enjoy it with an extra sprinkle of crushed walnuts and cherries or pour it into a bowl and eat it in true sundae style. Sub in any nuts or seeds instead of walnuts if you prefer.

1 cup unsweetened vanilla almond milk

1 cup frozen cherries

1 cup baby spinach

1 fresh or frozen banana

¾ cup plain or vanilla low-fat Greek yogurt

1 tablespoon walnuts or walnut butter

In a blender, combine all the ingredients and blend until the desired consistency is achieved. Add more liquid as needed. Serve immediately.

Bonus Boost:

Walnuts are one of the best plant-based sources of omega-3 fatty acids and can be helpful in reducing inflammation and pain.

Per serving:

Calories: 215; Total fat: 5g; Sodium: 143mg; Cholesterol: 5mg; Total carbs: 38g; Fiber: 4g; Sugar: 28g; Protein: 7g

LB's Blissed-Out Berries

Anti-Inflammatory, Heart Health, Immune Boost

SERVES 2

Bliss out with some of nature's top sources of natural fiber all in one glass. Berries and chia clearly share a seedy trait that makes them such great nutritional powerhouses. This simple purple blend calls for any type of unsweetened protein powder but feel free to sub in yogurt instead to balance out the carb and protein profile.

1 cup skim milk
1 cup frozen strawberries
1 cup baby spinach
½ cup frozen blueberries
½ cup frozen blackberries
2 scoops plain whey, pea, or hemp protein powder
1 tablespoon chia seeds

In a blender, combine all the ingredients and blend until the desired consistency is achieved. Add more liquid as needed. Serve immediately.

Per serving:

Calories: 242; Total fat: 3g; Sodium: 178mg; Cholesterol: 6mg; Total carbs: 32g; Fiber: 8g; Sugar: 12g; Protein: 23g

Pep in Your Step

Anti-Inflammatory, Brain Health, Heart Health, Immune Boost

SERVES 2

Step up your nutrition with this minty chocolate blend full of antioxidants, healthy fats, and fiber. Peppermint extract or mint leaves will leave you feeling fresh and ready to take on whatever the day brings your way.

1 cup unsweetened coconut milk

1 cup kale

1 fresh or frozen banana

¾ cup plain coconut yogurt

½ cup frozen raspberries

½ cup frozen coconut pieces

1 tablespoon chia seeds

1 tablespoon cacao powder

2 teaspoons peppermint extract or a few fresh mint leaves

In a blender, combine all the ingredients and blend until the desired consistency is achieved. Add more liquid as needed. Serve immediately.

Per serving:

Calories: 238; Total fat: 12g; Sodium: 126mg; Cholesterol: 0mg; Total carbs: 30g; Fiber: 9g; Sugar: 16g; Protein: 7g

Hair of the Dewy Dog

Anti-Inflammatory, Heart Health, Immune Boost

SERVES 2

Even when you're living a healthy lifestyle, it is normal to consciously indulge at times, so this smoothie is just what the doctor ordered to revive you after a rough night. Potassium-rich bananas, honeydew, and spinach combined with hydrating grapes and anti-inflammatory, spicy ginger make this mix a perfect hair-of-the-dog remedy. Try freezing grapes for a healthy snack or as a smoothie add-in.

1 cup unsweetened vanilla almond milk

1 cup baby spinach

1 fresh or frozen banana

¾ cup plain low-fat Greek

yogurt ½ cup honeydew

½ cup fresh or frozen grapes

1 tablespoon fresh ginger or 2 teaspoons ground ginger

1 tablespoon hemp seeds

In a blender, combine all the ingredients and blend until the desired consistency is achieved. Add more liquid as needed. Serve immediately.

Per serving:

Calories: 205; Total fat: 5g; Sodium: 152mg; Cholesterol: 6mg; Total carbs: 33g; Fiber: 4g; Sugar: 26g; Protein: 8g

Red Tango

Heart Health, Immune Boost

SERVES 2

Do the smoothie tango with a tantalizing twist of sweet vitamin C–rich mangos and fiber-boosting bloobs. Chia seeds and Greek yogurt add protein and filling fat to keep you dancing all day.

1 cup frozen mango

1 cup frozen blueberries

Handful baby spinach

1 tablespoon chia seeds

¾ cup plain 2 percent Greek yogurt

1 cup unsweetened almond milk

Combine all the ingredients and blend until desired consistency. Add more liquid as needed. Serve immediately.

Recipe variations

Dairy-free variation: Substitute plain coconut yogurt (Cocojune), pea protein yogurt (Ripple), almond milk (Kite Hill) or pili milk yogurt (Lavva) for dairy yogurt, or use plain pea or hemp protein powder.

Nut-free variation: Substitute dairy, hemp, oat, coconut, rice, or pea protein milk for almond milk.

Per serving:

Calories: 190; Total fat: 5g; Sodium: 149mg; Cholesterol: 6mg; Total carbs: 29g; Fiber: 6g; Sugar: 21g; Protein: 8g

Dr. Jeff's Cardiac Cocktail

Anti-Inflammatory, Brain Health, Heart Health, Immune Boost

SERVES 2

My brother is not only a top cardiologist but also has a heart of gold. His patients love him because even though he recommends a diet full of nutrient-dense fruits and veggies, he knows food has to taste good, too. This smoothie is chock-full of some of the best foods for your ticker. It combines fiber- and antioxidant-filled fruits and pomegranate juice with spinach and an omega-3–rich seed trio that knocks the heart -healthy nutrition out of the park. If you don't have pomegranate juice, you can omit it and increase the coconut milk to 1 cup.

1 cup watermelon

1 cup frozen mixed berries

1 cup baby spinach

¾ cup plain coconut yogurt

½ cup unsweetened coconut milk or coconut water

½ cup pure pomegranate juice

1 whole kiwi

1 tablespoon chia/hemp/flaxseed mix

In a blender, combine all the ingredients and blend until the desired consistency is achieved. Add more liquid as needed. Serve immediately.

Per serving:

Calories: 208; Total fat: 6g; Sodium: 126mg; Cholesterol: 0mg; Total carbs: 26g; Fiber: 6g; Sugar: 19g; Protein: 6g

Becky's Afterburn Boost

Anti-Inflammatory, Brain Health, Heart Health, Immune Boost

SERVES 2

For a post-workout refresh, blend up this mix of body-replenishing carbs and proteins with a boost of hidden cauliflower that will even satisfy Aunt Becky after her tough 6 a.m. spin workouts. Cottage cheese is another high-protein whole-food option for smoothie additions, so try it with a mix of sweet fruits for a sweet and salty combo that tastes good and provides an excellent balance of nutrition. Becky, your sore muscles will thank you tomorrow.

1 cup unsweetened vanilla almond milk

1 fresh or frozen banana

¾ cup plain low-fat Greek yogurt or cottage cheese ½ cup frozen mango

½ cup frozen blueberries

½ cup frozen riced cauliflower

1 tablespoon almond butter

1 tablespoon chia seeds

In a blender, combine all the ingredients and blend until the desired consistency is achieved. Add more liquid as needed. Serve immediately.

Per serving:

Calories: 270; Total fat: 10g; Sodium: 147mg; Cholesterol: 6mg; Total carbs: 38g; Fiber: 8g; Sugar: 25g; Protein: 10g

Raspberry Rainy Day

Anti-Inflammatory, Digestive Health, Heart Health

SERVES 2

Rain or shine, this red raspberry blend will do the trick to keep you full and satisfied. Packed with high-fiber berries and protein-rich yogurt, this sweet combo is as soothing as the pitter-patter of rain.

1½ cups frozen raspberries
1 cup unsweetened vanilla almond milk
1 cup baby spinach
¾ cup Siggi's whole-milk vanilla
yogurt ½ cup frozen pineapple
1 tablespoon chia seeds

In a blender, combine all the ingredients and blend until the desired consistency is achieved. Add more liquid as needed. Serve immediately.

Bonus Boost:

The enzyme bromelain found in pineapple is anti-inflammatory and has been linked to digestive health, so drink up.

Per serving:

Calories: 273; Total fat: 9g; Sodium: 165mg; Cholesterol: 14mg; Total carbs: 39g; Fiber: 10g; Sugar: 27g; Protein: 10g

Lola's Lemonade Stand

Brain Health, Heart Health, Immune Boost

SERVES 2

This smoothie is as sweet and simple as my daughter Lola's summer lemonade stand. Balance sweet strawberries and banana with sour lemons for a perfectly healthy lemonade treat with absolutely no added sugar.

1½ cups frozen strawberries

1 cup plain coconut yogurt

1 cup unsweetened coconut milk

1 fresh or frozen banana

¼ cup freshly squeezed lemon juice (about 3

lemons) 1 tablespoon chia seeds

In a blender, combine all the ingredients and blend until the desired consistency is achieved. Add more liquid as needed. Serve immediately.

Per serving:
Calories: 228; Total fat: 8g; Sodium: 136mg; Cholesterol: 0mg; Total carbs: 35g; Fiber: 7g; Sugar: 20g; Protein: 7g

Anna's Bananas

Anti-Inflammatory, Heart Health, Immune Boost

SERVES 2

Super-tart cranberries in a smoothie sound bananas but the combo of sour with sweet ingredients creates a balanced blend that tastes just like Ya Ya Anna's homemade banana bread. Cranberries, especially when consumed as whole fruit instead of juice, have a powerful nutritional profile high in plant compounds and antioxidants.

2 fresh or frozen bananas

1 cup unsweetened almond milk

1 cup baby spinach

¾ cup Siggi's whole-milk vanilla

yogurt ½ cup frozen cranberries

1 tablespoon hemp seeds Dash cinnamon

In a blender, combine all the ingredients and blend until the desired consistency is achieved. Add more liquid as needed. Serve immediately.

Bonus Boost:

Cranberries contain a tannin that helps prevent bacteria from adhering to the bladder and urinary tract, which supports kidney and bladder health.

Per serving:

Calories: 222; Total fat: 7g; Sodium: 132mg; Cholesterol: 12mg; Total carbs: 37g; Fiber: 5g; Sugar: 21g; Protein: 6g

Cha-Cha Cherry Chai

Anti-Inflammatory, Brain Health, Heart Health, Immune Boost

SERVES 2

You will wanna cha-cha through the kitchen when you get one taste of this sweet and soothing chai tea blend packed with cherries to create a delicious antioxidant stunner. You can cut open a chai tea bag and use the leaves instead of brewing it for even more taste and nutrition. If you don't have cloves, feel free to omit them or sub in nutmeg and/or ginger.

1 cup frozen dark cherries

1 cup baby spinach

1 fresh or frozen banana

¾ cup plain low-fat Greek

yogurt ½ cup brewed chai tea

½ cup unsweetened vanilla almond

milk 1 tablespoon ground flaxseed

meal Dash ground cinnamon

Dash ground cloves

In a blender, combine all the ingredients and blend until the desired consistency is achieved. Add more liquid as needed. Serve immediately.

Bonus Boost:

Cherries, spinach, chai, and additional spices are full of nutrients for heart health, and the combo of carbs and protein will keep your blood sugar stable.

Per serving:

Calories: 171; Total fat: 4g; Sodium: 118mg; Cholesterol: 6mg; Total carbs: 27g; Fiber: 4g; Sugar: 18g; Protein: 8g

Matcha Average Avocado

Anti-Inflammatory, Brain Health, Heart Health

SERVES 2

This blend is not your average green smoothie. Matcha (green tea powder) and avocado blended with blueberries and banana create a creamy mingling of antioxidant-rich, heart-healthy ingredients. Be on the lookout for frozen avocado at the market for your smoothie storage stash or use a fresh one. Either way, it will be avo you ever wanted to keep you full and satisfied.

1 cup unsweetened coconut milk

1 cup frozen blueberries

1 cup baby spinach

1 fresh or frozen banana

¾ cup plain coconut yogurt

¼ cup frozen avocado or ¼ fresh avocado 1 tablespoon hemp seeds

1 teaspoon matcha powder

In a blender, combine all the ingredients and blend until the desired consistency is achieved. Add more liquid as needed. Serve immediately.

Bonus Boost:

Matcha is high in catechins, a class of antioxidant that is thought to help fight cancer, so drink to your health!

Per serving:

Calories: 228; Total fat: 10g; Sodium: 132mg; Cholesterol: 0mg; Total carbs: 32g; Fiber: 6g; Sugar: 20g; Protein: 7g

Happy Holidaze

Anti-Inflammatory, Heart Health

SERVES 2

Whether it's that holiday time of year or not, this comforting but super-nutritious blend of ingredients will brighten up your day. Pure pumpkin is an underrated ingredient in any dish. It's one of the most economical, convenient, and nutritious ways to incorporate loads of vitamins A and C and beta-carotene into your diet for skin, eye, and heart health. If you don't have cranberries, you can omit them.

2 fresh or frozen bananas

1 cup unsweetened vanilla almond milk

1 cup kale

¾ cup Siggi's whole-milk vanilla

yogurt ½ cup pure canned pumpkin

¼ cup frozen cranberries

2 tablespoons rolled oats

1 tablespoon ground flaxseed

meal Dash ground cinnamon

In a blender, combine all the ingredients and blend until the desired consistency is achieved. Add more liquid as needed. Serve immediately.

Per serving:

Calories: 269; Total fat: 7g; Sodium: 127mg; Cholesterol: 12mg; Total carbs: 47g; Fiber: 8g; Sugar: 23g; Protein: 8g

Frozen Peanut Butter Hot Cocoa

Brain Health

SERVES 2

Inspired by the heavenly (but highly sugary) frozen hot chocolate from Serendipity ice cream shop in NYC, this version is a healthy treat that satisfies even the sweetest tooth but manages to do it without any added sugar. Garnish with mini chocolate chips, if desired.

1 fresh or frozen banana

1 cup unsweetened vanilla almond milk

1 cup frozen strawberries

1 cup baby spinach

½ cup plain low-fat Greek yogurt

2 tablespoons cacao powder

2 tablespoons peanut butter

Dash ground cinnamon (optional)

Mini chocolate chips, for garnish (optional)

In a blender, combine all the ingredients (except the optional chocolate chips) and blend until the desired consistency is achieved. Add more liquid as needed. Top with the chocolate chips (if using) and serve immediately.

Bonus Boost:

The powerful protein combo of peanut butter and yogurt will slow digestion, stabilize blood sugar, and keep you full and satisfied.

Per serving:

Calories: 249; Total fat: 12g; Sodium: 202mg; Cholesterol: 4mg; Total carbs: 33g; Fiber: 6g; Sugar: 18g; Protein: 10g

Secret Garden Smoothie

Anti-Inflammatory, Heart Health, Immune Boost

SERVES 2

It's no secret that veggies are the key for volume when it comes to a healthy diet. They fill your meals with tons of food and nutrition so you can eat more, but they are so low cal they help you naturally take in fewer calories. You've hit the jackpot in this medley because the double dose of veggies provides double the bang for your nutritional buck. When you blend them together with sweet mangos and banana, you will never know that there are carrots and zucchini in your cup, but your body sure will.

1 cup unsweetened vanilla almond milk

1 cup frozen mango

1 fresh or frozen banana

¾ cup Siggi's whole-milk vanilla

yogurt ½ cup fresh or frozen carrots

½ cup frozen zucchini spirals

1 tablespoon hemp seeds

In a blender, combine all the ingredients and blend until the desired consistency is achieved. Add more liquid as needed. Serve immediately.

Per serving:

Calories: 221; Total fat: 7g; Sodium: 123mg; Cholesterol: 12mg; Total carbs: 35g; Fiber: 5g; Sugar: 28g; Protein: 7g

Strawberry Shanny and Friends

Anti-Inflammatory, Heart Health, Immune Boost

SERVES 2

Life is not complete without your friends by your side, especially my bestie Shanny, who is always up for a good time. So, whip up this batch of strawberries blended with her other fruity friends for a party for both your taste buds and your health.

1 cup unsweetened vanilla almond milk

1 cup frozen strawberries

1 cup baby spinach

¾ cup plain low-fat Greek

yogurt ½ cup frozen pineapple

½ cup frozen peaches

1 tablespoon chia seeds

Dash ground cinnamon

In a blender, combine all the ingredients and blend until the desired consistency is achieved. Add more liquid as needed. Serve immediately.

Bonus Boost:

Full of antioxidants and fiber, this trio of fruit with spinach, chia, and yogurt is the perfect combo to keep you energized for a marathon shopping trip or anywhere your friends take you.

Per serving:

Calories: 158; Total fat: 4g; Sodium: 79mg; Cholesterol: 6mg; Total carbs: 26g; Fiber: 6g; Sugar: 17g; Protein: 7g

Roslyn Berry Blowout

Anti-Inflammatory, Brain Health, Heart Health, Immune Boost

SERVES 2

The moms in my suburban town of Roslyn love a good weekly hair blowout, so I jokingly refer to this smoothie as the Roslyn Berry Blowout. Its taste is so invigorating that it will make you will feel like you just stepped out of the salon with a fresh new 'do without ever leaving the house. A mix of high-fiber berries, potassium-rich banana, and spinach is a recipe for a great day in the neighborhood.

1½ cups frozen mixed berries

1 cup unsweetened coconut water or milk

1 cup baby spinach

1 fresh or frozen banana

¾ cup plain coconut yogurt

1 tablespoon chia seeds

In a blender, combine all the ingredients and blend until the desired consistency is achieved. Add more liquid as needed. Serve immediately.

Per serving:

Calories: 186; Total fat: 6g; Sodium: 58mg; Cholesterol: 0mg; Total carbs: 32g; Fiber: 7g; Sugar: 17g; Protein: 6g

Nat's Nutty by Nature

Anti-Inflammatory, Brain Health, Heart Health

SERVES 2

This berry banana smoothie includes a trio of heart-healthy nuts that stabilize blood sugar and provide lasting energy for a busy day. My smart dietitian friend Nat would explain that nuts are an excellent source of nutrition because they naturally contain all three macronutrients your body needs in one micro package. Sub in any nuts, seeds, or nut or seed butters for the ones listed in the recipe.

1 cup unsweetened vanilla almond milk

1 cup frozen raspberries

1 cup baby spinach

1 fresh or frozen banana

¾ cup plain low-fat Greek yogurt

1 tablespoon cashew butter

1 tablespoon almond butter

1 tablespoon walnut pieces

In a blender, combine all the ingredients and blend until the desired consistency is achieved. Add more liquid as needed. Serve immediately.

Per serving:

Calories: 295; Total fat: 11g; Sodium: 155mg; Cholesterol: 6mg; Total carbs: 34g; Fiber: 8g; Sugar: 19g; Protein: 14g

Kale 'Em with Kindness

Digestive Health, Heart Health, Immune Boost

SERVES 2

You don't know how many times I have asked, "Is there kale in my teeth?" I know, dietitians typically love and recommend kale, but it is for good reason. Kale is a nutritional superstar, full of a variety of vitamins, minerals, and antioxidants, which is why this leafy green works especially well in smoothies where it is mostly undetectable when paired with sweet fruits. Sub in yogurt or another protein powder if you don't have hemp protein.

2 cups kale

1 cup unsweetened vanilla almond milk

1 fresh or frozen banana

½ cup frozen mango

½ cup frozen pineapple

1 scoop vanilla hemp protein powder

1 tablespoon hemp seeds

In a blender, combine all the ingredients and blend until the desired consistency is achieved. Add more liquid as needed. Serve immediately.

Per serving:

Calories: 239; Total fat: 5g; Sodium: 189mg; Cholesterol: 0mg; Total carbs: 35g; Fiber: 6g; Sugar: 24g; Protein: 16g

Orange You Glad (This Is the Last Smoothie)!

Anti-Inflammatory, Brain Health, Heart Health, Immune Boost

SERVES 2

Orange you glad you bought this smoothie book? Me too! This filling blend of fruits and veggies hails from the orange family, which means it is full of vitamin C, potassium, and beta-carotene.

1 cup pure canned pumpkin or cooked sweet potato

1 cup frozen mango

2 mandarin oranges

¾ cup Siggi's whole-milk vanilla yogurt

½ cup unsweetened vanilla almond

milk 1 tablespoon chia seeds

Dash ground cinnamon

In a blender, combine all the ingredients and blend until the desired consistency is achieved. Add more liquid as needed. Serve immediately.

Bonus Boost:

Beta-carotene is found in orange fruits and vegetables and converts to vitamin A in the body, making it important for eye and skin health. Both you and eye will love this one!

Per serving:

Calories: 214; Total fat: 7g; Sodium: 89mg; Cholesterol: 12mg; Total carbs: 35g; Fiber: 9g; Sugar: 30g; Protein: 7g

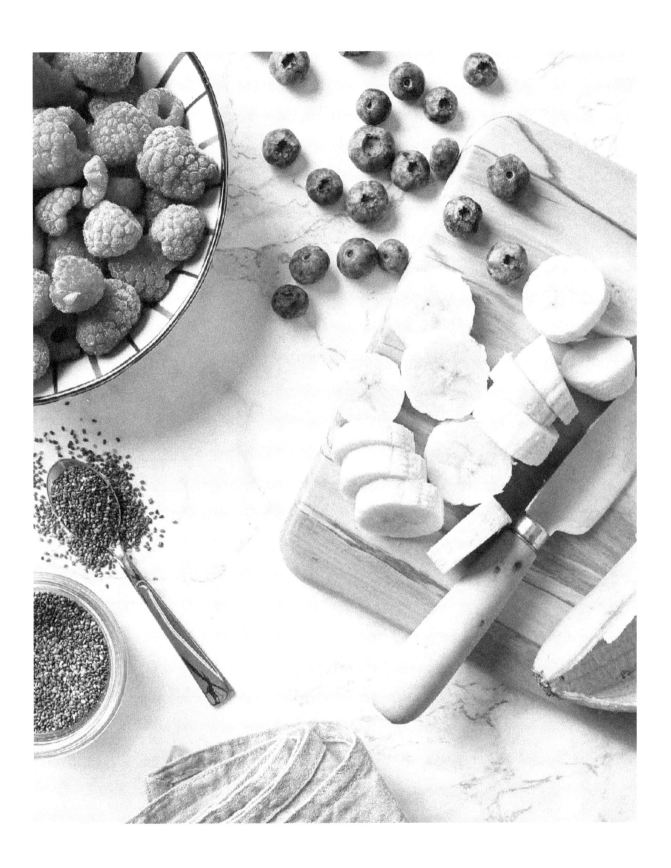

CPSIA information can be obtained
at www.ICGtesting.com
Printed in the USA
BVHW062131210621
610125BV00008B/2065